Dyslexia
and the Journalist

ALSO BY TONY SILVIA
AND FROM MCFARLAND

Robert Pierpoint: A Life at CBS News (2014)

*Fathers and Sons in Baseball Broadcasting:
The Carays, Brennamans, Bucks and Kalases* (2009)

*Baseball Over the Air: The National Pastime
on the Radio and in the Imagination* (2007)

Dyslexia and the Journalist

Battling a Silent Disability

TONY SILVIA *and*
SUZANNE ARENA

Foreword by Kate Griggs

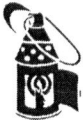

McFarland & Company, Inc., Publishers
Jefferson, North Carolina

All photographs without a source credited are from the personal collections of the authors.

Library of Congress Cataloguing-in-Publication Data

Names: Silvia, Tony, author. | Arena, Suzanne, author.
Title: Dyslexia and the journalist : battling a silent disability / Tony Silvia and Suzanne Arena ; foreword by Kate Griggs.
Description: Jefferson, North Carolina : McFarland & Company, Inc., Publishers, 2021 | Includes bibliographical references and index.
Identifiers: LCCN 2021032472 | ISBN 9781476682402 (paperback : acid free paper) ∞
ISBN 9781476642918 (ebook)
Subjects: LCSH: Dyslexia—Psychological aspects. | People with disabilities. | Journalism. | BISAC: LANGUAGE ARTS & DISCIPLINES / Journalism | SOCIAL SCIENCE / People with Disabilities
Classification: LCC RC394.W6 S55 2021 | DDC 616.85/53—dc23
LC record available at https://lccn.loc.gov/2021032472

British Library cataloguing data are available

ISBN (print) 978-1-4766-8240-2
ISBN (ebook) 978-1-4766-4291-8

© 2021 Tony Silvia and Suzanne Arena. All rights reserved

No part of this book may be reproduced or transmitted in any form or by any means, electronic or mechanical, including photocopying or recording, or by any information storage and retrieval system, without permission in writing from the publisher.

Front cover image © 2021 Shutterstock

Printed in the United States of America

McFarland & Company, Inc., Publishers
Box 611, Jefferson, North Carolina 28640
www.mcfarlandpub.com

Table of Contents

Foreword by Kate Griggs — 1
Preface by Tony Silvia — 3
Introduction by Suzanne Arena — 7

1. What Is Dyslexia? — 17
2. Images of Dyslexia in Media — 29
3. Fred W. Friendly — 42
4. Anderson Cooper — 57
5. Byron Pitts — 64
6. Robyn Curnow — 79
7. Gabrielle Emanuel — 95
8. Jill Wellington — 109
9. Richard Engel — 114
10. The Journalist's Role as Change Agent — 126
11. Resources for Journalists Covering Dyslexia and Disability — 141

Appendices
  A. "Millions Have Dyslexia, Few Understand It" by Gabrielle Emanuel — 151
  B. "Raising a Child with Dyslexia: 3 Things Parents Can Do" by Gabrielle Emanuel — 155
  C. "Dyslexia: The Learning Disability That Must Not Be Named" by Gabrielle Emanuel — 158
  D. Recognizing If Your Child Is Dyslexic — 161

Table of Contents

E. Fun Facts About Dyslexia   163
F. Famous Dyslexics in History   165
G. "5 Reasons Why Dyslexics Make Great Communicators" by Kate Griggs   167
H. Helpful Links and Resources on Reading   170
Chapter Notes   173
Select Bibliography   183
Index   185

Foreword

Kate Griggs

Right now, humanity is facing some of its greatest challenges—from a global pandemic to an escalating climate crisis. In this increasingly uncertain and unpredictable world, we need people who can make sense of the chaos. People who can look at the big picture and connect the dots. People who can pursue stories and causes with passion. People who can simplify a situation, or assess the facts and present an angle.

In this book, you'll find inspiring dyslexic journalists who do just that.

Take Byron Pitts, for example, whose grit and determination saw him overcome challenges at school to succeed on the world stage, winning Emmys for his coverage of events like 9/11 on CBS News. And Richard Engel, whose dyslexic strengths led him to connect the dots and explain the events of the Iraq War with insight and clarity, winning every award and accolade in his field—all after overcoming his own battles at school.

Many people may wonder why dyslexics excel in the field of journalism. But the answer is simple: the dyslexic brain is wired differently. We are highly skilled at communicating (71 percent of us are above average at it). This means we are able to connect stories and see patterns in narratives where others may not. Our dyslexic ability to simplify means we create clear and compelling messages. We're also able to use our high levels of empathy and emotional intelligence to connect deeply with the people whose stories we're telling. Many of us are also driven by a desire to create a better, fairer society.

That's certainly true at Made By Dyslexia. I've spent many years researching dyslexic strengths and made it my mission to help the world understand these strengths, through reports like *Spelling It Out*. I've collaborated with the global business consultancy firm EY to look at the

Foreword by Kate Griggs

game-changing power of dyslexia in the workplace. Together we produced the *Value of Dyslexia* reports, which pointed out that dyslexics have *exactly* the skills needed for the future world of work, as identified by the World Economic Forum. I've used my dyslexic strengths to create powerful and clear messages that drive change.

At Made By Dyslexia, our message couldn't be simpler: the world needs dyslexic thinking now. And we're making it our mission to empower dyslexic thinking in the future by training every teacher, and helping every workplace, to spot, support, and empower all dyslexics.

If communication is your dyslexic skill, or you're passionate about helping the world see dyslexia differently, I hope this book inspires you to share your story and make your voice heard.

This book is vital reading for anyone who wants to understand the bigger picture of dyslexia, journalists and readers alike, because in it, you'll meet bold, inspirational, and determined people who succeeded not in spite of their dyslexia, but because of it.

Kate Griggs is the founder and force behind Made By Dyslexia, a global charity led by successful dyslexics whose purpose is to help the world understand, value, and support dyslexia. Dyslexic herself, Griggs's "Creative Brilliance of Dyslexia" TED Talk led to the charity's groundbreaking Value of Dyslexia reports in association with EY, which demonstrate that, now more than ever, the future needs dyslexic thinking skills.

Preface

Tony Silvia

"Did you know there's a famous, legendary Rhode Island journalist who was dyslexic?"

That was my first question to Suzanne Arena in June 2019 on social media. I was struck by the fact that she founded an advocacy group called Decoding Dyslexia, RI, what I would later learn is a grassroots movement among parents, educators, and some enlightened legislators. Branches of Decoding Dyslexia are in all fifty states, four Canadian provinces, and, most recently, the continent of Africa.

All share a common mission: the fight for equal education for all children, through early testing and remediation of the most common learning disability in America, dyslexia.

Once we met and as I came to know Suzanne, I learned so much about her: her own undiagnosed dyslexia, her son Cole's learning difficulties related to dyslexia, and, most of all, her passion, commitment, and constantly evolving care and kindness for parents and children who have nowhere else to turn.

I've learned in our time together, Suzanne's and mine, that dyslexic children (and adults) constantly and consistently come out on the short end of the stick when it comes to public education. As you will read in the pages ahead, support for dyslexics is a catch-22. By that I mean in some states mandatory early testing exists, but forcing educators to do the right (and often legal) thing is still a battle.

Suzanne and her "warrior moms" (and some dads) have made enormous progress. As I came to be inspired by her mission (I won't call it a cause, because it really is a mission), I wanted to know more, to learn more about dyslexia.

Like most Americans, I thought dyslexia was a "thing" that some, though probably few, had. I thought it must be debilitating and

Preface by Tony Silvia

irreversible because, otherwise, why couldn't it be "cured" by using modern techniques in teaching reading? And wasn't it really all about, only about, seeing letters backward?

It was and still is an education for me, for someone who not only has a PhD, but also once studied education, including how to teach reading. It was an awakening.

I learned, through Suzanne and her strong band of sisters, that dyslexia is so much more than "reading backward." It encompasses a whole litany of allied behaviors that can contribute to additional learning disabilities, not to mention shame, low self-esteem, depression, and even self-destructive behavior in our children. I say "our" children because if we believe in an educational system (or if we say we do) where every child has an inherent right to excel, no matter the challenges they face, they are truly OUR children.

The legendary Rhode Island journalist to whom I referred was Fred Friendly. He truly was a legend, helping found what we now know as the medium of television news. Together with another legend, Edward R. Murrow, Mr. Friendly produced television programming that is today considered groundbreaking, historic, iconic, and world changing.

And he was also something in addition to a legend. He was dyslexic.

As our conversations continued, Suzanne and I decided to write an article about Fred Friendly, focusing on his accomplishments, despite (or maybe because of) his dyslexia. That article, repurposed here, was the foundation of the book you now have in hand.

Following conversations with Ruth Friendly, his widow, and Lisa Friendly, his daughter, we felt inspired to expand our research, asking ourselves, "Are there other journalists who navigated through their dyslexia to achieve at the highest levels in a field where the odds were stacked against them?"

We found there were, and we also found the results of our quest to discover what it is about dyslexia and journalism that makes the two more a "fit" than we might intuitively think. And if recognizable, celebrated journalists have dyslexia, we figured their stories could be a conduit for inspiration for others, children especially, who have similarly been told they aren't capable and should scale back their aspirations.

All of the journalists in our book were told that same thing, in some form, whether they were called "dumb," "lazy," or only suitable, in one instance, to be a wife or a mother, and, in another, labeled mentally retarded and recommended for institutionalization. One even recalls

Preface by Tony Silvia

having her teacher throw a book at her while using an epithet meaning "stupid."

As a journalist myself for over fifty years, as well as an educator, I know firsthand the power the media, the news media especially, have to influence perception, create awareness, and bring about change. If there was ever an area where change is not only needed, but also long overdue, it is in the images we have of those with dyslexia.

Those who are on the front lines of spreading information to the American public are in a unique position to educate, illuminate, and bring about that change—especially through telling their own stories as proof that, even in a field that is so steeped in reading and writing, the potential exists for every child, given the necessary support and resources.

Meeting Suzanne changed my way of thinking because, for one, I hadn't thought about dyslexia at all. Since then, I've done research and learned what it is, but more importantly what it isn't, how it may limit but also expand one's world. We may refer to dyslexia as an "invisible disability," while others (including several of the journalists in this book) call it a "gift."

In October 2019, I found myself giving a speech at the Rhode Island State House during Dyslexia Awareness Month. I've given hundreds of speeches over the years, but this is one I never expected to feel qualified to give. But in that moment, on a crisp fall day, I felt a strong pull toward a part of me I didn't know existed.

I felt a passion for those kids and their parents, many of whom were suffering silently and had been for a very long time. I felt a part of something bigger than myself. I began to embrace Suzanne's mission and that of Decoding Dyslexia. It is the worthiest of all missions.

We decided that the best way to approach our subject was to begin with Suzanne's personal journey. In the introduction to this book, I hope you sense the tapestry of a life lived with dyslexia, made so much more intense when left undiagnosed from childhood.

And the love between mother and son is everywhere evident in the bond between her and Cole. You'll find parts of her story heartbreaking, but that's the point.

Dyslexia can be heartbreaking, but it doesn't have to be. It can be affirming. It can be not a curse, but a gift. The word is "can."

Children (and adults) with dyslexia CAN.

And those outside of the dyslexic community can help by embracing them, by encouraging and providing the support needed

Preface by Tony Silvia

to make them full, visible members of our larger communities and schools.

Our hope is that you will be inspired by what you read, but also motivated to be better teachers, administrators, parents, and, yes, if this is your field, even better journalists.

People like Suzanne give tirelessly and without expectation of personal gain to help those who need it the most, as she says, "the kids."

We were all "kids" once, some of us more fortunate than others, but the voice we hear inside still calls out to help this generation and the next, by understanding *their* journeys.

Introduction

Suzanne Arena

> "It kills me that there are standardized tests geared towards just one kind of child."—Channing Tatum, actor

I grew up in Milton, Massachusetts, just fifteen minutes south of Boston. The schools were top rated in the 1970s and 1980s, and to this day Milton still holds the distinction of being in the top five best places in the United States to raise a family. That being said, I hated school. I often refer to myself as "the why child," because I am curious about everything and how it works. I can tell you if it wasn't for my art and chorus classes, I would have been invisible. Invisible because I was that child who stammered and stuttered when I was called on to read aloud and couldn't read what I was trying to focus on. I was put into tutoring, hated reading, and detested math.

Remembering the multiplication chart was not something I mastered … and then there was the dreaded periodic table, dates in history, capitals of states, and forget about learning the basic grammar, punctuation, and rules for our language. I admit that I was a quiet kid to everyone but my friends because I was afraid of being laughed at. My only saving grace was being known as the artist. I admit I cheated and developed an ability to deflect, although I really wanted to learn and was an avid reader of *National Geographic*; I studied the photos within its pages since I was first able to hold the magazine.

Among my most difficult memories was not being able to find my way around; I couldn't make sense of maps, and I must have had dozens of locks cut off my lockers (because I couldn't remember the combination) … but mostly I carried my books around with me. I typically enjoyed talking to older people and would listen to their stories for hours. I was told I was very smart in these situations and very kind. I never cared what others thought of me, and I always felt I was meant to

Introduction by Suzanne Arena

do something great, but I didn't know if that was writing books like Stephen King or Agatha Christie or inventing something. I was always having visions and coming up with ways to improvise and solve problems if something was broken or if I needed something. An adaptive problem solver is probably the best way I would describe myself.

The only secret most people didn't know about me was that I became a teen who engaged in self-harm. I had very low self-esteem and carried a lot of anger and sadness. I wrote poetry, which I only shared with my English teacher, Mrs. Currier, who said that my gift was intense ... but my story was tragic; she wanted me to keep writing and keep a diary. I did, and when I was fourteen, I took hundreds of pills to get out of my house and seek escape. I didn't care if I went into a foster home, I just needed to get out of my desperate situation. I didn't. The situation only got worse. However, it was around then that I decided I wanted to be an art therapist or do something to help children with trauma through art, and I worked really hard and read book after book, and that year things changed. I eventually was admitted to a community college, and my first quarter I made the dean's list. For the first time in my life I was soaring. But the reading became too much, and I was living on my own, plus working. I regret dropping out of college because I couldn't keep up with the work.

I didn't know then, or for many years later, that my mounting problems in school and with navigating life could be summarized in one word. That word is dyslexia.

Years later I married and at thirty-eight gave birth to my son, Cole. One of the greatest achievements and a great source of pride for parents is seeing and hearing their child read to them. For me, that moment didn't come until Cole was very far into fifth grade. My first-born child didn't know many of the letters in the alphabet, a fact that I came to realize when Cole's kindergarten classmates knew letters of the alphabet and their numbers cold.

First grade was next. All the students in the class were reading, but my child wasn't. Instead, he was still saying baby words; others often would say how "cute" it was when he used "words" like "albabet," "Stupermarket," or "pasketti." Cole was that child who couldn't tie his shoes, tell time, or understand other concepts that his school peers easily achieved. My very kind, thoughtful, and terribly sweet little boy was incredibly smart outside of his struggles in school.

I recall going to school during a parent-teacher night and looking at the class reports strung sloppily on a string with clothes pins. I

Introduction by Suzanne Arena

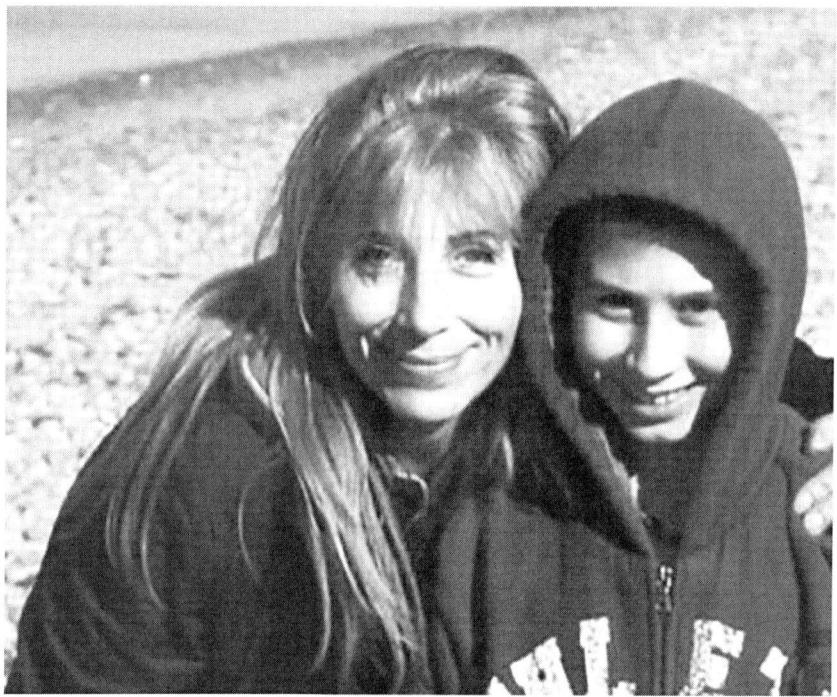

Suzanne Arena and her son, Cole, 2012, when Cole was in fourth grade.

am the type of person who likes to look at all the children's work, and the theme was based on what would you like to be when you are older. Most kids chose fireman, movie star, doctor, etc., but when I came to my son's I couldn't read the writing and looked up at his picture of an astronaut with his little face pasted on the head. It reminded me of *The Little Prince*, only his body was huge, floating on the little lost planet. I suddenly became very aware of others near me peering to look at his work, and I wanted to cry. I wanted to cry because he had struggled so hard to write, and, when frustrated, he would erase so hard that the paper would tear. He had tried to do this report in his best writing. I had seen the heavy concentration it took for him to write, but it still was mostly illegible. I intuitively knew something was wrong. I recalled the days of daycare when he would uncharacteristically act out and throw books or push over the bookcase. One time he even gave himself an injury from a bookcase falling on him, requiring stitches in his head.

I had Haven Miles (LCSW), with 30 years of experience, and she was the supervisor of Early Childhood Services at the Providence

Introduction by Suzanne Arena

Center, go into the daycare Cole attended to observe and then work with him. I also had him involved in the mental health program at Bradley Pediatric Partial Daycare. This was a four-week program, so I had to take a short-term leave of absence from work. The conclusion of both of these interventions was that he was underdeveloped in coping. They didn't have a name for what he was going through, so they came up with that. I told them I had a forty-two-year-old at home (my then husband), who also had coping issues. My question for the experts: Do they ever learn? I didn't know that Cole had a far more serious problem. I recalled even before then that he had colic in his first year of life, as well as chronic ear infections, in addition to extreme sensitivity to sound, touch, and taste. I learned over time, in talking with other parents, that these were common afflictions in dyslexic children.

My son's younger sister was already reading some words in kindergarten, and Cole was still eagerly attempting shoe tying, along with lots of other tasks that were laborious and often sent him into tantrums. As I compared sibling milestones and recognized Cole's learning was behind, I began to see the problem and began spending more time studying the issue. Some of the other differences between my son and the other kids were explainable because I read that boys developed slower; so, I was patient. I read every book I could such as *Oppositional Defiant Behavior*, *ADHD*, *The Angry Child*, etc. I left their dad when the kids were just five and six, so I didn't know if some of the behaviors could be attributable to that breakup. In first grade, his teacher agreed with me that there was something awry, and she suggested going to the doctor to look into his impulsivity. They ended up diagnosing him with attention deficit hyperactivity disorder (ADHD), and I tried a year of several medications, leading to tears and weight loss. I ended up taking him off medication when he was eleven, after he fainted and said his heart was jumping out of his chest. I saw no reason for this because he didn't display problems when he was home.

Looking back, I now know the joy of reading is an impossible achievement for one in five American children who are struggling as undiagnosed dyslexics ... it makes sense now that I know all the research, but it was devastating at the time. Reading is not natural and must be taught. However, communication is natural. There had to be a way to merge communication with reading, and that became my mission.

All this time, I watched my child struggle through the early grades. He received classroom remediation through the federally recognized

Introduction by Suzanne Arena

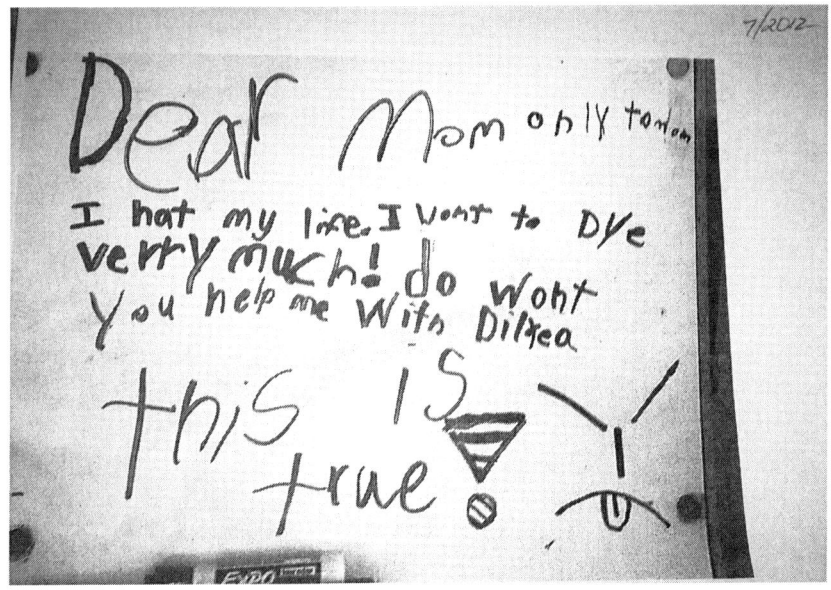

Cole Arena, at ten years old, wrote on his whiteboard that he wanted to die.

program Response to Intervention (RTI), and had a personal literacy program (PLP).[1] I would spend hours upon hours on the internet researching and trying to learn what my child's problem was, and while doing so, I came across a book that mirrored so many of his issues. The book, *Overcoming Dyslexia* by Dr. Sally Shaywitz, was truly an "A-ha!" moment.[2] I wanted to learn why my third grader was reading at a first-grade entry level. I became that warrior mom determined to educate myself, network, and advocate for my child. I heavily studied the laws and regulations, only to learn that schools must be compliant. I encouraged parents and students to take Pete Wright's boot camp training or utilize his website.[3] The schools hadn't identified my child for a suspected specific learning disability (SLD),[4] which I found out they are obligated to do under the Child Find Mandate.[5] The last straw for me was the day when my ten-year-old painfully drew on his white board easel, which usually was something creative and beautiful for him. Instead, he wrote "Dear Momoniy to MoM ... I hat my life, I vont to Dye very much! Do wont you help me with Dilxea ... this is true!" That was when I realized I needed to spend the $1,500 to have him tested for dyslexia.

The ironic part is the school said they couldn't test for dyslexia; although it is a specific learning disability, they said it was a medical

Introduction by Suzanne Arena

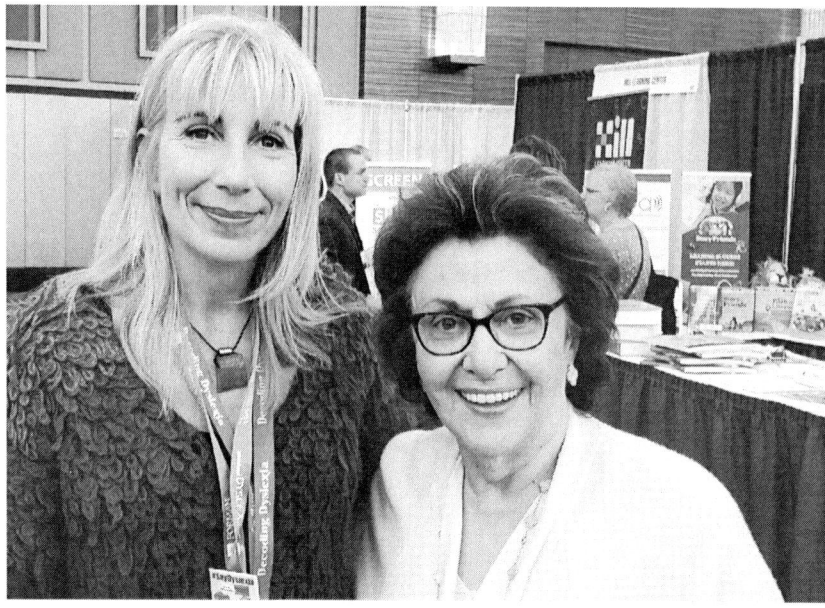

Dr. Sally Shaywitz, reading specialist scientist and co-founder of Yale Center for Dyslexia & Creativity (right), and Suzanne Arena, 2018.

versus an academic issue. We then went to a neuropsychologist who told us it was really an educational issue and the schools should be testing and covering these costs. It's a conundrum. It still is for most parents of dyslexic children.

I went through years of only getting two to three hours of sleep because I was mentally in crisis due to my child not being able to read and being grade levels behind. I agonized that he didn't have access to the education every child deserves, and I couldn't afford an attorney, so I decided to read and learn as much as I could to fight the school and their attorney. We were outgunned. During the summer after he graduated from third grade, I had Cole tested for a potential learning disability because the school was doing nothing and, at this point, I was pretty sure it was dyslexia.

The report came back and validated he not only had dyslexia but dyscalculia (math language challenge), dysgraphia (handwriting disability), low working memory, and ADHD. I remember being outside in the car when they were at the playground later that day and feeling overwhelmed, and tears quietly ran down my cheeks as I now knew not only what was wrong with my son, but also what had been wrong with me. I

Introduction by Suzanne Arena

was undiagnosed and suffered, and so much of what I had experienced mirrored with my child. He wasn't stupid, nor was I. I felt relief and validation. I knew at that point I better put on my armor and get ready to battle.

When Cole was twelve years old, in 2014, I was on the internet and stumbled on Decoding Dyslexia, a grassroots organization led by volunteer parents who had established themselves in many states. Soon after, I established the Rhode Island branch of Decoding Dyslexia in 2015, and this grassroots nonprofit provided support and guidance to parents in crisis. I fought to get my son what he needed to learn using a methodology known as the Orton-Gillingham method.[6] One of my main goals was to get legislators to pass a dyslexic bill to help our children receive the tools they needed. During that time, I had a parent and teacher, Kari Kurto from Texas, reach out to me and share she was moving to Rhode Island. She taught at Rawson Sanders, a dyslexia school in Texas where student achievement was attained through implementation of accredited multisensory structured language education, and she intended to stay within our community.[7]

I was incredibly grateful for her insights as a teacher. We shared the same passion and purpose, to give dyslexic children the ability to learn in ways they could understand, to provide them with accommodations that would unlock their hidden gifts further enabling them to soar and go on to be successful in life. At that time, I didn't think my child would or could ever go to college. Frankly, I didn't see much of an opportunity for him to have a great career because he was between a first- and fourth-grade reading level. Kari worked with me, and eventually, together with two other parents, we formed a group with a board of directors and put together what became known as the "dyslexia bill" that would (1) define dyslexia and require the "experts" to use the word dyslexia when making a diagnosis; (2) mandate screening in grades 1–3 to identify at-risk readers; (3) give teachers professional development to learn about signs, symptoms, and appropriate remediation; and (4) remediate only through evidenced-based systematic learning.

That first year we couldn't get the bill passed in the Rhode Island legislature, and schools were still not using the "D" word. However, during the next legislative session, we pushed hard using social media, holding rallies at the Rhode Island State House, and calling into radio talk shows, in addition to doing interviews. We became one of the top ten states to pass this important legislation, even though we were initially met with a wall of resistance in the Rhode Island Senate. Part of

Introduction by Suzanne Arena

that was because I decided to go to the local newspaper and was fortunate to meet a seasoned journalist, who heard my alarm and recognized that all of these lost kids needed to have their voices heard; she did a personal story about my son with a strategic rollout of the story on the front page of the *Providence Journal*, three weeks before the Senate would have to vote on the bill.[8] The article's pressure worked, and we were grateful to the journalist. The bill was then passed and signed by Rhode Island's governor in June 2016.

Ironically, the governor's son has dyslexia; she had pulled him out of Providence public schools and placed him in the only dyslexic private school in the state, named the Hamilton School at Wheeler, when he was nine years old. Fast forward to June 2019 when we were able to get additional legislation passed, and we continue to press ahead. We have worked with the Department of Education with a new commissioner, who also has a dyslexic child.

It's important to keep in mind that teachers are not trained in the science necessary to actually teach children how to read, as we'll discuss in detail in the next chapter. Horrifying, I know! Therefore, children who are most at risk are not having their needs met. It was an amazing public admission to have validated what we had been saying for a long time. What is the solution for teachers? One answer is to have universities actually teach them how to teach kids to read as opposed to letting them guess. Recently, the education journalist Emily Hanford[9] has been reporting on and exposing what she has labeled the Reading Wars.[10] It has been widely heard and circulated on public radio and elsewhere.

For the last eight years I have been a self-appointed volunteer parent advocate to help parents in crisis navigate the system. Those were some of my darkest years, during which I had the opportunity to speak to dyslexic children who were feeling worthless, to others who wanted to have a career as a teacher, writer, actor, doctor, engineer, news reporter, governor, etc. I have also spoken to parents who have children who are hospitalized with paralyzing trauma from this process. Among the things we would like students to know is this: if you see a child who is a paralyzed but doesn't have a wheelchair, that child is handicapped and incapable of going to school to access their education. However, if they are given the accommodation like that wheelchair, they can then access what they need to achieve their dreams. It's the same for a dyslexic child. If we do not provide the means, call it a vehicle or whatever accommodation is needed to access a full education, we are discriminating against whole generations by not allowing them to achieve. We need

Introduction by Suzanne Arena

students to not feel shame, be lost, or feel invisible because we send the message through our actions (or inactions) that their opinion doesn't matter.

This book is an opportunity to allow future generations to know the possibilities that exist for them and to send the message that anything is possible, especially with grit and grace helping you work through your challenges. Recently, there was a national survey on what our youth want to be when they grow up. In our home state of Rhode Island, most children chose the job of journalist. So yes, you can be a journalist, even if you are dyslexic. You can be just like the high-achieving journalists in this book. I am so in awe of these amazing people whose personal journeys you will read about. They have courageously shared their stories with us, in the hope of helping our children in the dyslexic community grow, evolve, and see the myriad opportunities that lie ahead in their lives.

Everyone needs strong role models, and it is our hope that parents, children, students, and practicing journalists will find inspiration in reading these stories of perseverance, strength, and accomplishment, often in the face of staggering odds against them achieving in a field centered around reading and writing skills. Our purpose is to present their stories in a manner that shows not only who they are, but also what *you can be*. For students and practicing journalists, we have the additional hope that you will learn more about dyslexia and how best to approach covering what we call "the invisible disability." You will read advice from each of the journalists profiled, but also gain insight into what we sometimes call "best practices" in researching, interviewing, writing, and presenting issues related to dyslexia. While our focus is on dyslexia, on a broader scale, our purpose is to improve the images, appreciation, and representation of all disabilities in our news and entertainment media.

Just as so few teachers are trained in how to teach reading to dyslexic children, few journalists are schooled in how to report on disability. In most instances, journalists have learned enough in school or in practice to cover stories about people who are blind, deaf, or paralyzed, but dyslexia remains a mystery to many reporters and editors. In writing our book, we want to demystify and "decode" or unlock the important questions about dyslexia you may have as a student sitting in a journalism class or as a professional who has never approached the subject. We focus on the childhood experiences of those profiled in the pages ahead, but remember, there are a lot of undiagnosed adults out there too … and it's never too late to go back to school! Learning never ends,

Introduction by Suzanne Arena

and these celebrated journalists, who shape the perceptions of millions of Americans (and millions more abroad), play a major role in fostering understanding of the issues that face us—be they cultural, political, environmental, medical, or educational. As such, they—and you in your role as a journalism student or a seasoned journalist—can do good or harm, depending on how authentically and accurately you tell the stories of the dyslexic community.

It is reassuring to know we have luminaries like Anderson Cooper, Richard Engel, Robyn Curnow, Byron Pitts, and Gabrielle Emanuel, among the others profiled here, who are part of and give back to our community. The probability is high that you know a dyslexic child or adult—even if you don't know you do. Don't only teach but learn from her or him. Welcome them into your circle because they have a lot to give.

As Byron Pitts of ABC News said to us, "What does a dyslexic look like?" He or she looks just like "us." There is no visible identifier. That makes it difficult for the general public, as well as journalists, to fathom a condition so common and yet so invisible. Take the time to explore, accept, and learn from these stories. Our goal and purpose is that, by the end of this book, you will understand a little more about what Robyn Curnow, one of those profiled here, calls "the gift of dyslexia." It is that gift of understanding that we give you now. Thank you in advance for accepting it!

Chapter 1

What Is Dyslexia?

> "Dyslexia is not a pigeonhole to say you can't do anything. It is an opportunity and a possibility to learn differently. You have magical brains, they just process differently. Don't feel like you should be held back by it."—Her Royal Highness, Princess Beatrice

> "If anyone ever puts you down for having dyslexia, don't believe them. Being dyslexic can actually be a big advantage, and it has certainly helped me."—Richard Branson, Virgin CEO

When you think of dyslexia, does the idea of someone reading "backward" or flipping their letters and numbers come to mind? You're not alone, because that's how most people think of dyslexia, but the reality is it's so much more. First you should know it's a spectrum with varying levels of learning challenge severities. You should also know that, whether you are a dyslexia expert or far from it, it's very easy to be fooled by the misinformation that surrounds the "D" word. Conclusion: people's individual experiences with dyslexia are as unique as their fingerprints.

The most prevalent types of dyslexia make it hard to match individual sounds with written symbols, missing connecting words like the, an, a, on, and, etc. This causes difficulty in one's ability to learn. Throughout this book you will hear similar experiences among journalists who have found ways to compensate using alternative methods of learning. Increased awareness is needed to reveal the truth about dyslexia. The goal is public understanding of this very common condition.

According to the International Dyslexia Association and the National Institutes of Child Health and Human Development, dyslexia is defined as:

> a specific learning disability that is neurobiological in origin. It is characterized by difficulties with accurate and/or fluent word recognition and by

poor spelling and decoding abilities. These difficulties typically result from a deficit in the phonological component of language that is often unexpected in relation to other cognitive abilities and the provision of effective classroom instruction. Secondary consequences may include problems in reading comprehension and reduced reading experience that can impede growth of vocabulary and background knowledge.[1]

Here in the twenty-first century, dyslexia still isn't given the recognition or awareness it is due among pediatricians, schools, mental health providers, doctors, and the public. We have the scientific research to know better, but we still don't do better. Dyslexia is listed in the *Diagnostic and Statistical Manual of Mental Disorders* (DSM-5 diagnostic code 315.00), which is a manual for assessment and diagnosis of mental disorders used by psychiatrists. Although the manual does not include information for treatment or guidelines to address dyslexia, it has become an alternative term referring to a pattern of learning difficulties characterized by problems with accurate or fluent word recognition, poor decoding, and poor spelling abilities. The specific learning disorder with impairment in written expression includes possible deficits in spelling, grammar, punctuation, accuracy and clarity, or organization of written expression. A comorbid challenge for some dyslexics is math, which is diagnostically labeled as dyscalculia and is also in the DSM-5.[2]

First let's look at pediatricians. They have a responsibility to identify milestones reached or any anomalies in what is considered normal. Pediatricians are a valuable partner; however, we need our pediatric practices to be empowered in ensuring their physicians have an ability to treat, educate, and advocate for their patients and families with dyslexia. It is especially important that they understand and highlight evidence-based and practical strategies for the implementation of early risk identification.[3]

This dyslexia diagnosis is what parents seek out from neurologists or other qualified professionals. Public schools are not required to test for dyslexia, but they are obligated to test to find out if a child is eligible for special education services, and if so, under what category. Children are being denied the necessary testing, and parent frustration is at a high point because they know for their child to receive the necessary services, they must have a diagnosis. Therefore, we say the data drives the program needs. So, parents privately seek independent evaluations knowing the schools lack the knowledge to recognize the characteristics of dyslexia. Alternatively, many parents feel it is budgetary and schools are intentionally not identifying children.

Chapter 1. What Is Dyslexia?

What can parents do when their child is failing, but no action is being taken at school? You should know that federal regulations state unequivocally that parents of a child with a disability have a right to obtain an independent educational evaluation (IEE).[4] An IEE is broadly defined as "an evaluation conducted by a qualified examiner who is not employed by the public agency responsible for the education of the child in question." Parents can obtain an IEE at public expense as explained later in this article.

It is important to note that an IEE is not limited to evaluating only a child's academic or cognitive skills, but may also include the evaluation of any skill related to the child's educational needs. Neurological functioning, sensory needs, aquatics, even music therapy are but a few types of IEEs covered under the Individuals with Disabilities Education Act (IDEA, 20 U.S.C. §1400[c][5][B]).[5] Parents may obtain an IEE for virtually any purpose if it impacts the child's education. The value of an IEE is to provide and strengthen the role of parents in the educational decision-making process.

Unfortunately, data reported as to the number of children being diagnosed with dyslexia and other comorbid disabilities varies because there is no universal definition of dyslexia. Parents stumble in the dark and learn the hard way. Among the lessons is their child must be tested by a neurologist, a licensed educational psychologist, or some other qualified medical professional to get a diagnosis. However, the schools are only required to "consider" the diagnostic report; they also can ignore it.

The paradox for parents is when they feel their child has a learning disability, which they believe is dyslexia, but it has never been identified by the school. In some public schools, when a child is struggling with the signs and symptoms of a learning disability, it becomes the parents' responsibility to pressure the school to test their child. However, the schools often respond that they can't diagnose for dyslexia because it's a *medical* issue, and therefore it's on the parents to seek a medical professional. This testing involves a long waiting list.

Misconceptions and myths about dyslexia are plentiful. Dr. Nadine Gaab[6] of Boston Children's Hospital and Harvard Medical School has an excellent presentation on "The Typical and Atypical Reading Brain: How a Neurobiological Framework of Reading Development Can Inform Educational Practice and Policy," which reflects some of the world statistics on diagnosing dyslexia.[7] Schools currently require repeated failure before students can even be considered for evaluation. We know

Dyslexia and the Journalist

teachers are not taught about dyslexia while earning their teaching degree; therefore they cannot identify early signs of dyslexia, such as deficits in phonological awareness, rapid automatized naming, verbal working memory, and letter knowledge, which have been shown to be robust precursors of dyslexia in children as young as age three.[8]

Dr. Gaab's research within the Laboratories of Cognitive Neuroscience focuses on the brain correlates of reading development in typical and atypical children as well as possible early signs of developmental dyslexia in preschoolers and infants. Dr. Gaab is a pioneer using functional magnetic resonance imaging (fMRI), a noninvasive brain imaging tool, as well as behavioral measurement tools to study the reading brain in infants and preschoolers, which is ongoing to date. Another study shows there are clear differences in brain mapping of dyslexics and nondyslexics, in that the children with dyslexia had greater functional connectivity from the left inferior frontal gyrus seed point to the right inferior frontal gyrus than did the children without dyslexia.[9]

A recent study of more than 1,200 kindergartners in New England not only identified six independent reading profiles, including three dyslexia risk profiles, but also showed that these reading profiles are remarkably stable over a two-year window (Ozernov-Palchik, in press). Furthermore, studies involving brain measures, such as electroencephalography or magnetic resonance imaging, have shown that the brain characteristics of individuals with dyslexia can be *observed as early as infancy and preschool*, especially in children with a genetic risk for dyslexia.

A longitudinal dyslexia study in Finland, which followed children from birth until age eight, showed that early differential brain measures could distinguish at-risk children who later developed reading problems from those who did not. "Dyslexia—Early Identification and Prevention: Highlights from the Jyväskylä Longitudinal Study of Dyslexia" concludes that there are numerous measures that can predict a child's potential for later difficulty with literacy.[10] However, from a practical perspective, the most salient indicators of later difficulty lie with expressive language delay and delay in acquisition of the names of letters, and a plethora of speech and language measures (e.g., physical activity, rapid naming, family literacy environment) that exert an influence on a child's later difficulty. It is suggested that close attention should be paid to children who display delayed language and/or who may not be grasping the letters of the alphabet in line with expected developmental milestones.[11]

Would you be shocked to learn that teacher training at universities

Chapter 1. What Is Dyslexia?

doesn't include learning the practical skills needed to teach children how to read? The problem is that even teachers who are trained in special education are not taught how to teach reading. While the science on reading was settled four decades ago, future teachers are still not being taught the appropriate and proven methodology, hence the battle continues. The outcome is that far too many teachers graduate with insufficient training in their field.

The public expects elementary teachers to be qualified to teach reading. There is a very specific set of techniques that has been around for forty years, and yet far too many of our teachers, through no fault of their own, are not prepared to deliver. That has led to some prominent elected officials and other experts nationwide to comment that we are denying our dyslexic children a basic right to learn. It could be argued that children are discriminated against by not providing those with disabilities the necessary tools to access their education under what is known as free and appropriate public education (FAPE).[12] It would be difficult to find teachers who are knowledgeable about dyslexia, let alone even say the word. Therefore, the comorbid learning disabilities like dysgraphia, dyscalculia, low working memory, and attention deficit hyperactivity disorder (ADHD), are anomalies. Parents not only trust schools with their children's education and welfare, but believe educators are experts because they have college degrees. Nationwide, the parent grassroots movement called Decoding Dyslexia has publicly exposed that teachers attending universities are *not* given the necessary training. Thousands of parents volunteer and advocate for their child's right to be taught to read.

These parents discovered their child is slow with processing reading, comprehension, fluency, math, etc., and have learned their undiagnosed child is neither getting identified nor being given the appropriate remediation. Signs of breakdowns include tantrums, headaches, and gastrointestinal problems, or twitching and ticks. These can lead to anxiety, depression, and other mental health, social, and emotional issues, which can be eliminated if dyslexics receive the same evidence-based reading instruction, but with intensity and repetition to help them map words by recognizing them with automaticity. It's hard to fathom that we began to discover reasons for learning problems a little over a century ago, yet most parents still have to fight for equal opportunities and appropriate education. Below is a brief timeline that tracks the history of learning disabilities from 1877 to our recent laws and scientific findings.[13] After viewing the timeline, ask yourself, how can dyslexia continue to fall at the bottom of the literacy continuum in our educational institutions?

> **1877**—The term "word blindness" is coined by the German neurologist Adolf Kussamaul to describe "a complete text blindness ... although the power of sight, the intellect and the powers of speech are intact."
> **1887**—The German physician Rudolf Berlin refines our definition of reading problems, using the term "dyslexia" to describe a "very great difficulty in interpreting written or printed symbols."
> **1895**—The ophthalmologist James Hinshelwood describes in the medical journal *The Lancet* the case of acquired word blindness, where a fifty-eight-year-old man awoke one morning to discover that he could no longer read. Hinshelwood continued to study word blindness in children and recognized the need for early identification of these children by teachers.
> **1896**—After reading Dr. Hinshelwood's report, Dr. W. Pringle Morgan writes in the *British Medical Journal* about a fourteen-year-old Percy F. who seemed to have word blindness from birth. He was the first to describe dyslexia. He says Percy "has always been a bright and intelligent boy, quick at games, and in no way inferior to others of his age. His great difficulty has been—and is now—his inability to learn to read." Percy "had great difficulty reading and spelling despite the efforts of his teachers. The schoolmaster who has taught him for some years says that he would be the smartest lad in the school if the instruction were entirely oral."
> **1905**—The first U.S. report of childhood reading difficulties in the United States is published by the Cleveland ophthalmologist Dr. W. E. Bruner. The term "dyslexia" wasn't commonly used in the United States until the 1930s.
> **1955**—The Food and Drug Administration (FDA) approves the drug Ritalin for treatment of depression and fatigue, but not for ADHD. (ADHD won't be recognized by the medical community for another thirteen years.)
> **1961**—Ritalin is first used to treat "hyperkinetic" symptoms in kids.
> **1963**—Samuel A. Kirk, a psychologist in Chicago, is the first person to use the term learning disability at an education conference.

Chapter 1. What Is Dyslexia?

- **1964**—The Association for Children with Learning Disabilities (ACLD) is created. They are now known as the Learning Disabilities Association of America (LDA), and there are chapters in every state.
- **1968**—Congress passes the first federal law requiring support services for children with learning disabilities.
- **1969**—Congress passes the first federal law mandating support services, known as the Children with Specific Learning Disabilities Act. This act is included in the Education of the Handicapped Act of 1970 (PL 91–230).
- **1973**—Congress passes Section 504 of the 1973 Rehabilitation Act. It bans discrimination against people with disabilities in programs receiving federal funding, including public schools.
- **1975**—Congress passes the Education for All Handicapped Children Act (EAHCA) (PL 94–142), which requires public schools to provide "free and appropriate public education" (FAPE) for all students. (This law is renamed the Individuals with Disabilities Education Act in 1990.)
- **1977**—The National Center for Learning Disabilities (NCLD) is formed by Pete and Carrie Rozelle.

The U.S. trends during the 1980s and 1990s reflect medical and education communities striving to understand learning disabilities and ADHD, and also how to help people who have them. Today, ADHD has become a more widely known term, but there is controversy about kids being over diagnosed.

- **1987**—A report released by the Interagency Committee on Learning Disabilities calls for the establishment of the Centers for the Study of Learning and Attention, whose sole purpose is to expand research and understanding of this issue.
- **1990**—The Individuals with Disabilities Education Act (IDEA) renames and changes the EAHCA (PL 94–142). The term "disability" replaces "handicap," and the new law requires transition services for students. Autism and traumatic brain injury are added to the eligibility list.
- **1996**—Dr. Guinevere Eden and her research team at the National Institute of Mental Health use functional magnetic resonance imaging (fMRI)—a process that allows us to look at the activity in living brains—to identify the regions of the brain that behave differently in dyslexics.

1997—IDEA is reauthorized. Regular education teachers are included in the IEP process, students have more access to the general curriculum and are included in statewide assessments, and ADHD is added to the list of conditions that could make a child eligible for services under the category "other health impairment."

2004—IDEA is reauthorized again. School personnel now have more authority in special education placement decisions, and the new law is better aligned with the No Child Left Behind Act (NCLB).

2005—Dr. Jeffrey Gruen and his research team at Yale University identify a gene that has patterns and variations strongly associated with dyslexia.

Although the U.S. federal government became involved in learning disabilities through task forces, legislation, and funding during the 1960s and 1970s, learning disabilities are not a new concept in the study of scholastic difficulties; its roots can be traced back to the early 1800s.[14] The earliest believed recognized case of a learning disability occurred in 1802, when Franz Joseph Gall, a German-French anatomist and physiologist and Napoleon's surgeon, recognized an association between brain injury in soldiers and subsequent expressive language disorders.

Studies show that individuals with dyslexia process information in a different area of the brain than nondyslexics. One can look at the historical research before 1900, when dyslexia was described as "word-blindness."[15] There have been a number of studies and research on this topic, but they have not reached institutions of education.

The United States has had a serious problem of ignoring the science and data for decades. Dyslexia *is* a serious problem and one deserving of instructional attention. The term dyslexia has been controversial and consequently has been avoided by most reading educators and special education teachers for decades.

In the 1980s and 1990s, a new method of teaching reading called whole language emerged and took over, replacing phonics.[16] This whole language theory is harmful to young children, as its advocates believe that learning to read and write English is analogous to learning to speak.[17] Further, whole language believers feel that reading is a natural, unconscious process; however, opponents of this theory counter that this is totally contradictory to the science because reading is not natural for humans.[18]

Chapter 1. What Is Dyslexia?

Most would be shocked to discover that teacher training at universities doesn't include learning the practical skills needed to teach children how to read. We need all teachers entering the school system, especially those in special education, to be taught about the signs and symptoms of learning disabilities and to know the methods in which children are taught to read. While the science on reading was settled four decades ago, future teachers are still not being taught the appropriate and proven methodology. The outcome is that far too many teachers graduate with insufficient training in their field, and these children are the ignored illiterate elephants in the room.

A parent uproar over children failing has turned the tide against standardized tests.[19] Professors are quick to share how these kids are not ready for college when they graduate high school and still need remedial instruction. The last five decades have fueled what has been described as "the reading wars," pitting "phonics-based" instruction against "whole language" instruction.[20] Basically, teachers moved away from systematic phonics instruction, words study, and comprehension strategies, allowing students to memorize text without learning reading strategies. This mixture of phonics-based and whole language instruction is known as balanced literacy and has emerged in the last decade. As long as educators are free to hold differing opinions, then this centuries-old debate will continue.

> "If your goal is to get little kids to reading comprehension, you want to work off their language comprehension, and teach them how to read those words. They know the meaning of lots of words, but not how to read them."—Emily Hanford

Emily Hanford has been reporting for a decade now on the deep-rooted problems with our education system, and 2019 was pivotal in the news across the country.[21] Hanford has been working in public media for more than two decades as a reporter, producer, editor, news director, and program host. She went to American Public Media (APM) in 2008 to produce documentaries for American Radio Works, which became part of APM Reports in 2016. A simple Google search of her name returns a plethora of articles, interviews, podcasts, etc., focusing on related outcomes due to our inadequacies in teaching those to read and how it affects our incarcerated population, creating a lack of qualified job candidates, along with mental and medical issues. She has been a powerful voice defining not just the origin of the problems but providing clearly mapped solutions.

Dyslexia and the Journalist

Until we start giving children the appropriate methods to learn based on science grounded in evidenced-based outcomes, children will succumb to educational malpractice. Data repeatedly supports early reading proficiency as vital to a child's ability to thrive both academically and mentally, as evidenced in the Annie E. Casey Foundation important study, "Students Who Don't Read Well in Third Grade Are More Likely to Drop Out or Fail to Finish High School."[22] In the final analysis, dyslexia is not just an educational problem, but it also constitutes a serious public health concern to our society.

So, what can you as an aspiring journalist do to help create awareness about an invisible disability? If you are aspiring to make a career in journalism, here are some qualities you should have, all of which can help you in deciphering not only dyslexia, but a whole range of learning disabilities.

- A way with words
- Thorough knowledge
- Investigative skills
- Effective communication skills
- Professionalism and confidence
- Persistence and discipline
- Ethics

There are many other specific qualities that a journalist who reports on any community, including those with disabilities, should strive to possess.[23]

1. **Curiosity:** A good journalist must be curious about all things. He/she must always be questioning the world in which he/she lives in.

2. **Honesty:** A journalist must be an honest person by nature, as there is no room in journalism for manipulation and/or lies. The truth is the truth. A journalist must look at the world objectively, but not too objectively that it hinders his/her ability to think critically.

3. **Fearless:** A good journalist must not be afraid. He/she will be in situations where tough questions must be asked. He/she might be in the middle of physical danger. A journalist cannot be afraid of taking risks and/or adventure.

4. **Loyalty:** A good journalist must be loyal. He/she must always keep in mind his/her job's purpose as a journalist: to be the public's watchdog. A journalist must always do his/her job for the good of the public's interest.

Chapter 1. What Is Dyslexia?

    5. **Kind:** A good journalist must be kind. He/she deals with different people daily, whether it be sources, coworkers, or state or national officials. A good journalist must be kind, unless someone warrants it to be any different.
    6. **Trustworthy:** A good journalist must be a trustworthy person. When building relationships with sources, these people will only help a journalist when they know he/she can be trusted.
    7. **Passionate:** A good journalist must be passionate about what he/she does. It's this passion that can make an impact.
    8. **Tenacious:** A good journalist must have a sense of tenacity. A good journalist cannot be discouraged easily, but rather thrive off the challenge.

Here are some other tips that you should keep in mind while reading the personal stories of those journalists with dyslexia in the pages ahead. As you learn about their journeys, consider the qualities of a good journalist that they possess.

What Makes a Good Journalist?

A good journalist must be resourceful. Resourcefulness gives a person the ability to always find a solution to difficult situations that can otherwise be at a dead end. Dyslexic students grow up learning how to cope and create workarounds when faced with something they can't seem to overcome. They must be committed and have great work ethic, which later proves to be most important. This is where many aspiring journalists have problems, and this is no doubt why someone with dyslexia would be able to do well in this career because they develop "workarounds" and have the perseverance to be resourceful. Often, they must develop strategies with highly complex thinking to succeed at accomplishing a task, and being a lateral thinker and problem solver provides an enormous advantage over others.

Dyslexics have an intrinsic ability to "scan," meaning they don't get caught up in the small details of a story, instead focusing on the most important aspects. The difficulty with phonetic decoding is a hallmark characteristic of dyslexia, often leading to the practice of scanning. This is why most dyslexia remediation focuses so heavily on phonics. It makes sense to intensify instruction in the area where the student seems to struggle the most. While this approach helps dyslexics see things from every angle, it is a huge advantage for journalists. Additionally, being

Dyslexia and the Journalist

able to make creative leaps of thought opens up innovative approaches to storytelling. Often referred to as a "Why Child" in school for his or her thirst to understand, the dyslexic student learns to ask questions in ways that give him or her a solid understanding. These children learn to keep asking until they get the answer they require—again, a valuable quality for any journalist.

Many of the journalists whose stories you will read in the following pages echo what many dyslexics and their parents know all too well. Most were not identified in school; they didn't get the help they needed to be successful; they were bullied and made to feel dumb because the signs and symptoms of dyslexia were unknown to them. After so many decades, there is a major need to ensure that our children don't needlessly suffer the way we did. As you'll see in these stories, the journalists profiled have amazing perseverance, a strong work ethic, and the grit to be the best advocates they can be for those whose voices have been silenced for too long.

For so many in America and around the world, all they know about people who are different from them is learned not from textbooks, but from mainstream and streaming media. The media's voice can be both powerful and destructive in terms of creating either accurate representations or misrepresentations of various groups in our society. Dyslexics have both benefited from and been harmed by their representation in television, motion pictures, and news coverage, as we shall examine in our next chapter.

Chapter 2

Images of Dyslexia in Media

"Whoever controls the media, the images, controls the culture."—Allen Ginsberg, poet

"All media exist to invest our lives with artificial perceptions and arbitrary values."—Marshall McLuhan, philosopher

The Importance of Media Representation

Positive media representations of people with any disability are critical in terms of improving the self-image of those in the community affected. Studies have shown that positive portrayals in media can impact one's self-image, self-esteem, self-motivation, and overall well-being. The theory of media effects basically reinforces this idea that there are social and psychological effects that result from the interaction between media and individuals, communities, or small groups, and that those effects can either be positive or negative.[1] Media can have the "effect" of sending messages that suggest a strong range of possibilities or a dead end for those in the affected group. The impact directly relates to the individual or group's perception that success is possible or that failure is inevitable.

There are several possible outcomes or effects that result from seeing one's self represented in a positive versus a negative manner. The often unintended consequences of media messages can have the effect of enhancing an individual or group's sense of self-realization or hampering it. On one hand, one's potential for achievement and success in a career, in life, or simply in connection to others both inside and outside the group or the community hinges on strong, positive or at least accurate and nuanced (rather than stereotypical) representations of

Dyslexia and the Journalist

those who are part of that group. On the other hand, no representation in media of a group leads to invisibility and ultimately, as is often argued in connection with racial and ethnic groups (Native Americans, especially), a concept referred to as symbolic annihilation.[2] In the simplest terms, if people from a certain group or community never see themselves represented, there is a sense of "I don't exist" or matter to anyone in the larger society.

It has become accepted that "for many community groups and organizations, gaining positive and consistent coverage in the media can have an incredible impact on the work they do." There are many reasons for this, but, according to one group, "it can have a multiplier effect on the good work that groups are doing. If people know what you have achieved and what you do, they are more likely to support your group. The more support you get, the more likely you are to have a bigger impact." That study's conclusion: "While it is important that groups don't become obsessed about getting media attention as a bigger priority than actually doing the work they do, it can make a difference."[3]

This is true for many with disabilities. In the instance of dyslexia, many dyslexics absorb and process information less from the written word than from depictions in popular visual media, television and movies, especially. Until relatively recently, young people with dyslexia had few, if any, role models in popular entertainment media to provide the range of their potential for achieving in school, the workplace, a profession, or simply as people with true value to others in society. There are exceptions, in all forms of media, but that's the problem: they are exceptions. They stand out because the message can become that they are not the norm; rather, they add to the narrative that those with disabilities—in this instance, dyslexia—are different. They are the "others," not "us." The narrative often suggests, in its subtext, that they are to be celebrated, but that they are not "typical" of others with the same condition. For any marginalized group, representation on a broad scale is a major component of self-awareness, self-value, and self-actualization. This is certainly the case for young people with dyslexia, during the most formative period in their lives.

The media landscape has changed enormously since the advent of the internet. Streaming services have a major influence on the viewing habits of today's youth, but television, both broadcast and cable, maintains considerable influence over the images and portrayals of disability presented to both children and adults. Dyslexia, while we have called it the "invisible disability," has nevertheless been in the spotlight of several

Chapter 2. Images of Dyslexia in Media

popular sitcom and dramatic series, some of which include historically highly viewed programs.

For example, as early as the 1990s, the network soap opera *General Hospital* included a character named Stone Cates, who was dyslexic. While this was groundbreaking for its time, the character also had a short life. Stone Cates represented more of a plot device, a way to inspire the other characters on the show by overcoming his challenges.[4]

Even earlier, in 1989, NBC's *The Cosby Show* featured Cosby's TV son Theo (played by Malcolm Jamal Warner), one of the first characters on television to openly struggle with dyslexia. The character is said to have been based on Cosby's own son, Ennis, who was dyslexic. For several seasons, Theo is shown struggling with his dyslexia. In what has been called a "landmark episode," titled "Theo's Gift," he is depicted studying hard and learning new ways to improve his grades. In the final episode, Theo graduates from New York University with a psychology degree. The writer Susan Corsall has observed similarities between the two young male characters—Stone Cates and Theo Huxtable:

> Both were portrayed as teenage boys who teachers and parents thought simply did not apply themselves. The boys themselves struggled and believed that they were stupid. That was until they were diagnosed with dyslexia and given the help they needed. The portrayals seemed to accurately depict the struggle of the boys, but I don't recall any of the tools or strategies they used being shown on a regular basis. Stone used a sheet of colored plastic to assist him in reading words when he was first diagnosed, but then it seemed to disappear. Often times, it seemed as if after the character was introduced with dyslexia and their struggle was explored in that episode, [but] it wasn't mentioned again. Thus, television has portrayed dyslexia positively in that it has shown that it does not mean that the student is stupid and that it is something they can receive help with.[5]

Alternatively, the fact that dyslexia was viewed as a short-term disability that could be confronted and cured quickly, in the space of a thirty-minute sitcom or soap opera, belies the reality that dyslexia is not easily "fixed." Outside of television, most dyslexics struggle for years without the opportunities or resources to improve and thrive. Both characters, and the others we will discuss, also present a version of dyslexia that is "one size fits all," characterized by reading difficulties: the stereotypical "seeing backward," reversing letters. As we've shown above, dyslexia takes many forms, reading among them, but other variations include math and trouble with following directions.

In 2005, the popular ABC drama *Grey's Anatomy*, at this writing in

Dyslexia and the Journalist

its seventeenth season, featured a high-achieving dyslexic doctor, Cristina Yang, who was diagnosed with dyslexia at age six. The story line didn't reveal this, however, until season four, when viewers learned that Cristina got straight A's throughout medical school; much is made of her perseverance, which is reinforced in every episode. It has been pointed out that the show's writer, "instead of just keeping Cristina as a driven woman who turned to medicine ... she also made the character dyslexic. Being dyslexic can be especially difficult for developing children, but most people can overcome the disorder and lead normal, professional lives." Again, however, dyslexia is a character development device; "they didn't go over her dyslexia much in the series, but it is just another back story detail that makes her character all the more compelling."

Corsall suggests this may represent progress, nonetheless, in terms of positive images of dyslexia on TV. Of the Yang character, she states, "This reaffirms my belief that some shows may use a dyslexia ratings boosting story line and then abandon it. Having watched the show many times, I figure I missed that episode because I never realized Cristina Yang was dyslexic. Maybe this is good because they are portraying her as a successful doctor who has overcome her learning disability. However, this can also be seen as an unrealistic portrayal in that she doesn't have to cope with the struggle of the disability on a daily basis."

Several other representations of dyslexics on television include:

* *The George Lopez Show* (ABC, 2002–07): Pivotal here is an episode in which George faces difficulty in accepting his son, Max, as dyslexic—but even harder is the realization that he may be too. This presents a scenario that actually mirrors real life, wherein a parent discovers the same symptoms of dyslexia in themselves as in their child, a not uncommon occurrence.
* *Beverly Hills 90210* (ABC, 1990–2000): The character Donna Martin doesn't do well on her SATs and thinks her college dreams are over. Instead, it's discovered that she has dyslexia, and she takes the test over as an oral exam, doing much better, and ultimately attends college. Notable is the fact that a 1991 episode "marked one of the first times accommodations for dyslexia were talked about on TV."
* *My So-Called Life* (ABC, 1994): The character Jordan Catalano reverses letters when he writes and is not a good student overall. One episode is titled "Why Jordan Can't Read," in which he balks at the idea that he is dyslexic, instead insisting, "Hey, I can

Chapter 2. Images of Dyslexia in Media

read, OK? I'm just not that good at it." Interestingly he is good at songwriting, so the message sent is that dyslexics are capable of other things beyond formal classroom learning. In many ways, it was a breakthrough.

Another positive role model for young people with dyslexia was the Disney Channel's *Shake It Up* (2010–13). Bella Thorne, who played Ce Jones, represented a rarity in any form of media: an actress with a disability playing a character with a disability. Ce Jones, the character, is dyslexic and the actress playing her is also dyslexic in real life. "Dyslexia might have made things more challenging, but it didn't stop me, and the challenge made me stronger," Thorne has said.

While *The Tonight Show* on NBC is in a different genre than any of the programming discussed above, its former host, Jay Leno, has presented a strong image for those with dyslexia. During his two decades on the air and since, Leno has openly spoken on multiple occasions about his own experiences with dyslexia. He has even used it as material for his comedy, citing his stern Scottish mother who emigrated here to the United States as a child. "My mom was a smart lady, but certainly not a well-educated lady, so she put a lot of effort into education," he says. "But when you're dyslexic and your mother has a Scottish accent and she's trying to teach you fourth-grade French, there's nothing funnier," he once said in an interview. Beyond the laughter, Leno has also insisted over the years that *difference* doesn't have to quell ambition, even in a difficult field like television. "I discovered that being a little bit different actually sets you aside in show business; it makes you special," he says. "You always try to turn your negative into a positive."[6]

One study suggests that, from 1984 to 2013, at least fifteen characters in sitcom or dramatic series were represented on television as "dyslexic." Only four, the study found, were female, which does represent the scientific reality that more boys than girls are *diagnosed* as dyslexic. That's because boys more often act out in school. That doesn't mean, however, that girls don't have it.[7] Whether there was intent to represent that fact accurately or there are simply more male characters on television than female characters is difficult to assess.

In some television sitcoms, the tendency has been to play dyslexia "for laughs," an unfortunate occurrence because it suggests ridicule, rather than support. As one observer put it, "In comedy, it's usually portrayed as jumbled, hilariously misspelled words, sometimes used in order to spell rude words—if spelling something incorrectly a dyslexic wouldn't necessarily form recognizable words at all."[8]

Of course, television is only one medium that has an effect on how dyslexics are viewed by the broader society. Movies also occupy a central place in popular culture and exert a major influence on how people view others like them—or not like them. Because of the cross-effect of theatrical movies being eventually aired on television and through streaming services, their impact is intensified. Together with documentaries, much progress has been made in the depiction of those with dyslexia, in fact, more so than what we have seen in the medium of television.

Dyslexia in the Movies

While there have been several movies portraying dyslexia in the entertainment genre, the majority of media images are contained within documentaries. A fair number of documentaries focus on dyslexia, often as a form of inspiration to those inside and outside the dyslexic community. Several are noteworthy due to their influence through distribution on subscriber cable and streaming services like HBO. All present a personalized approach to the topic of dyslexia, which is less "one size fits all" and more in the realm of spreading enlightenment on the complexity of those with dyslexia.

Dyslexic herself, E. S. Peck, a film critic for the website "Reel Rundown," is in a position to judge the efficacy of documentaries in conveying authentic images of dyslexia. "For most people, watching a documentary is an easier way of picking up information than reading a book," she writes. "For many dyslexics, this format is an ideal way to learn more about themselves, and connect with others who face similar challenges."[9] She cites four documentaries that were most effective in helping her cope with her own dyslexia.

The first is *Like Stars on Earth*, an Indian film depicting a boy whose troubles in school are magnified by the fact that he is undiagnosed as dyslexic. He meets an art teacher who recognizes visual skills and abilities other educators failed to notice. Peck writes that "this film did an amazing job of demonstrating the natural creativity that many dyslexic individuals exhibit, and how much good concentrating on those areas does. It also shows the unique pain of being unable to perform in a traditional setting, the fallout resulting from repeated failure and the exclusion felt by those who don't fit in."

Chapter 2. Images of Dyslexia in Media

At the same time, as with many media representations of dyslexia (and other disabilities), the film also has its share of stereotypes surrounding the dyslexic child needing to be "rescued" by an astute, caring teacher (an occurrence that does exist in real life, as you will read in the profiles of those we interviewed, but, sadly, is not the experience of all dyslexic children). As Peck puts it, "the story line was a little clichéd, too. There are so many stories floating around where one particular teacher saves a struggling student, that I feel kids might expect someone to come save them, when that rarely happens."

Next is *Embracing Dyslexia*, a 2013 film that shares the first-person stories of those living with dyslexia. It does so by interviewing dyslexics, from students to adults, at different points in their lives, leading up to their eventual successful professional careers. Peck's assessment is that "*Embracing Dyslexia* does an amazing job of demonstrating the emotional impact of how people treat dyslexics when they're younger and the strengths it gifted them with. It also highlights how important it is to get intervention early in life. At the end of the film, he includes some extremely good suggestions about how to improve the culture in which our children grow up."

Don't Call Me Stupid is a British documentary, aired on the BBC and produced by actress Kara Tointon, herself dyslexic. In the film, she emphasizes lesser known challenges posed by dyslexia, such as memorization and organizational skills. "This documentary is unique in that it addresses the problems of the adult dyslexic," according to Peck. "People tend not to realize that dyslexia never goes away, and its effects linger throughout a person's life. However, *Don't Call Me Stupid* demonstrated opportunities grown dyslexics may not realize they have."

Best known, and perhaps most influential due to its prominence on HBO, is *The Big Picture: Rethinking Dyslexia*. Showing the full range of possibilities for those with dyslexia, this film features interviews with parents and children impacted by dyslexia, as well as a surgeon, lawyer, and politician who are dyslexic. Most notable is the presence of Richard Branson, who relays his own personal strategy for combating the short-term memory problems experienced by many dyslexics—making lists of ideas before board meetings to ensure he didn't forget major points.

In Peck's assessment, "It was wonderful to see people of all ages represented, and to see how it affects people in unexpected ways outside of the classroom. Two of those ways that hit a cord with me was the impact of poor quality of handwriting, and how frustrating combination locks on lockers are. I still have nightmares of being unable to get into my locker in high school." This, too, while not being universal, is the reality faced by many dyslexics and, as such, presents an accurate image. Their power is not in their perfection, but in their *presence*. Collectively, they create a media space where dyslexics can see themselves and experience inclusion, rather than the ostracism many experience in their daily lives. "Although there's no such thing as a perfect documentary, these four films do wonderful jobs of addressing different aspects of the unique struggles people with dyslexia face on a regular basis," concludes Peck.

Some of these films appear on other critics' lists of those where dyslexia is either a topic or the focus. There are others that have been labeled as "inspiring." Manprett Singh assembled and annotated such a list in 2019.[10] It includes a 1985 film titled *Love, Mary*, based on the real-life story of a dyslexic teenager who went on to "beat the odds" and become a medical doctor. Her earlier life consisted of a trip to reform school for disruptive behavior, where a counselor sees her potential and helps build her self-confidence and study skills. Again, there is this thread of someone coming to a dyslexic's "rescue."

This is also a theme in the 1981 film, *The Princess and the Cabbie*. The plot revolves around a heroine, Joanna, who accidentally meets a cab driver wanting to help her overcome her dyslexia. The cabbie helps Joanna with her struggles in reading and writing, after finding a book she left in his cab. The plotline can only be described as contrived, but the attempt to help a dyslexic girl by an ordinary, nonexpert citizen is laudable, if not representative of reality.

Similarly, *Anya's Bell* (1999) depicts a blind woman who accidentally meets a twelve-year-old delivery boy who is, at first, a "slow learner," but later discovered to be dyslexic. Each helps the other with their struggles, the boy learning Braille and each progressing toward increased self-reliance and independence. Inspiring, yes, but again, the plot falls short of reflecting the daily challenges faced by most, or at least many, dyslexics.

More realistic is 1992's *The Secret*, notable also because it is rare to see a major Hollywood star, in this instance Kirk Douglas, play a major role in a film about dyslexia. A drama, the story line shows an authentic side of many dyslexics: their shame and reluctance to tell anyone about their learning disability. The main character is an older adult with dyslexia, who struggles with reading and writing, but is too proud to reveal his "secret" to anyone. The turning point comes when he learns that his grandson suffers from dyslexia as well.

Chapter 2. Images of Dyslexia in Media

Finally, *A Mind of Her Own* (2006) is based on another true story about a young girl who wants a career in medicine, but whose parents think a different career would suit her better, due to her severe dyslexia. Sophie instead perseveres, and, with the help and encouragement of her friend, puts herself through college and achieves her dream.

While all of these films are enriching and inspiring, they also fit the description of what has been referred to as "inspiration porn"—stories that inspire those with disabilities to *believe* they can achieve through good old-fashioned persistence and perseverance. It's a familiar media narrative, but how closely does it track reality? Does it give people with disabilities hope or false hope? What role does "inspiration porn" play in terms of the lens through which those with disabilities are viewed? Does it help or hurt? And who is it intended to most inspire—those with the specific disability portrayed or the larger society, by creating a "feel good" aura around those who might otherwise make us feel uncomfortable? These are important questions for *all* in the disability community. They are especially important to those with dyslexia. Because those with dyslexia receive less of society's attention than those who are blind, deaf, or paralyzed (all clearly visible and identifiable forms of disability), the authenticity of narratives primarily designed to "inspire" others takes on special significance.

The Media and "Inspiration Porn"

In 2012, the Australian comedian, writer, and social activist Stella Young coined the term "inspiration porn" to describe media narratives that depict those with disabilities as being not ordinary, but extraordinary, based on the idea they could accomplish a task beyond their own and society's expectations. As she puts it, "Inspiration porn is an image of a person with a disability, often a kid, doing something completely ordinary—like playing, or talking, or running, or drawing a picture, or hitting a tennis ball—carrying a caption like 'your excuse is invalid'" or "before you quit, try."[11] The inspiration arises from the concept that these "special" people serve to inspire others with the same disability, along the lines of "if he/she can do it, why can't you? Try harder, persevere more, and you can make it, too." Social media was largely responsible for spreading the use of the term, in particular a TED Talk that Young did in 2016, months before her death.[12]

In that talk she made a number of salient points about how media and society approach stories surrounding disabilities in general; all apply to those with dyslexia. When the intent is primarily to inspire, the result can often be an unrealistic portrayal of an entire group, making it seem as if everyone in that group is the same. It may also involve the kindness of an outsider toward the challenged individual. There are many examples in news coverage, among them the high school wrestler who gave up his perfect season to let a Down syndrome opponent win.[13] Others include the severely autistic students elected homecoming king and queen of their high school.[14] Many of these "inspirational" narratives go viral and center on the image of a disabled individual who prevails in life primarily, if not *only*, due to the help of an "abled" person. These narratives can take on the aura of universal truth. This fulfills a need for the nondisabled community. Think back to the earlier part of this chapter and how many dyslexic adults and children in the movies achieved their dreams only through the kindness of an "abled" teacher, counselor, or someone else who, ultimately, drove that success.

In her initial article on the topic, Young writes: "Let me be clear about the intent of this inspiration porn; it's there so that nondisabled people can put their worries into perspective. So, they can go, 'Oh well, if that kid who doesn't have any legs can smile while he's having an awesome time, I should never, EVER feel bad about my life. It's there so that nondisabled people can look at us and think 'well, it could be worse…. I could be that person.'"

The harm, she suggests, is in the images of disabled people as those who are either extraordinary on their own (rare) or got to where they are with help from others (frequent): "In this way, these modified images exceptionalize and objectify those of us they claim to represent. It's no coincidence that these genuinely adorable disabled kids in these images are never named: it doesn't matter what their names are, they're just there as objects of inspiration. But using these images as feel-good tools, as 'inspiration,' is based on an assumption that the people in them have terrible lives, and that it takes some extra kind of pluck or courage to live them. For many of us, that is just not true."

Young cites an "inspirational" photo of a paralyzed girl drawing a picture using a pencil she's holding in her mouth, suggesting that much of inspiration porn involves children or young people doing what other "ordinary" kids do, but making it seem special. "That's the thing about those kids in the inspiration porn pictures, too—they're not doing anything their peers don't do," she writes. "We all learn how to use the bodies we're born with, or learn to use them in an adjusted state, whether

Chapter 2. Images of Dyslexia in Media

those bodies are considered disabled or not. So that image of the kid drawing a picture with the pencil held in her mouth instead of her hand? That's just the best way for her, in her body, to do it. For her, it's normal."

As the originator of the term, Young attributes a good number of the false narratives involving all disabilities to the media and to journalists in particular. "I can't help but wonder whether the source of this strange assumption that living our lives takes some particular kind of courage is the news media, an incredibly powerful tool in shaping the way we think about disability." She concludes that "most journalists seem utterly incapable of writing or talking about a person with a disability without using phrases like 'overcoming disability,' 'brave,' 'suffers from,' 'defying the odds,' 'wheelchair bound,' or, my personal favorite, 'inspirational.' If we even begin to question the way we're labeled, we slide immediately to the other end of the scale and become 'bitter' and 'ungrateful.' We fail to be what people expect."

One might ask what harm there is in providing people with hope through inspiration. Doesn't that, in the process, at least create and spread awareness? Even if the narrative is nonrepresentative of those with a disability, doesn't it have shared value anyway?

Eileen Daly, another critic of inspiration porn, argues that the harm, not the value, is strong. She cites a video that trended on Twitter in early 2019. It depicted a bride and groom dancing at their wedding. However, what made this wedding unique was the groom is in a wheelchair and was helped by two guests to stand and complete the dance midway through. Videos like this are harmful, Daly argues. "In this example, the bride and groom are simply objects for the benefit of nondisabled people. The couple is being used to motivate able-bodied people to reflect on how lucky they are. But disabled people do not exist in order to inspire and motivate the able-bodied population."

Daly challenges the assumptions we make about all forms of disabilities. "As you watch the video, what are you thinking? Is your first thought, Gosh, the beautiful bride is a hero to marry someone like him? Why are able-bodied people seen as heroes simply for treating disabled people as human beings? Disabled people date. We have sex, we fall in love, we get married. We have kids, some get divorced. Some of us are sporty, some of us are not…. Conversely, not all disabled people are good or saintly. Having a disability does not make me a morally righteous person. We make mistakes, we fail sometimes, we are human." The real harm, she concludes, is that "inspiration porn is the objectification of one group of people to make another group feel better about themselves."[15]

Additional harm results from the internalization of the message to some disabled people that "you're not good enough because you can't do what others like you can do." As Saidee Wynn suggests, "Inspiration porn also ignores the fact that there are many different types of disabilities and perpetuates the assumption that disabled people should be able to do anything. This is just not true."[16] She concludes that it puts an undue burden on those with disabilities to be an inspiration in order to "matter" to the rest of society.

This ignores the fact that race, education, gender, and socioeconomic realities are all factors influencing access to the kinds of resources needed to help people live with a disability. All disabled people are not alike, just as all *people* are not alike. To suggest that a dyslexic child can "overcome" his reading, writing, math, or motor skills difficulties just by "trying harder," becoming more motivated, or paying increased attention in school is a false narrative. However, it's one that's forced on many people with other disabilities. It's even more so forced on dyslexic people because of the assumption in American society that everyone can read if they really want to. So those who can't are called lazy or stupid. This is a reality faced by all of the journalists we profile in this book.

The disability advocate Kit Mead suggests that a by-product of inspiration porn is that it "portrays people with disabilities as 'others'—less than human, or a lower level of human. Because we are 'other,' acts of kindness toward us seem newsworthy."[17] Alternatively, Amy Lutz argues that the real story resides in the act of kindness, not the disability, and that's where the inspiration is generated. She writes that

> acts of kindness—significant gestures that reflect thought, consideration, and concern—are newsworthy, period. It doesn't matter whether one of the parties is disabled or not. Take the story of the Alabama college student who mowed the lawns of the elderly in his neighborhood for free, or the African American college student who brought Starbucks treats to white police officers. Or the employee at a Georgia Wal-Mart who literally gave the shoes off his feet to a homeless man. Or the members of a football team from a California high school, who each dropped an orange rose at the feet of a cheerleader suffering from leukemia.

All of these, she suggests, demonstrate "a need to see more kindness in the media, not less."[18]

Bringing the conversation back to our major topic, a solution may reside in those journalists who are themselves dyslexic, not only battling

Chapter 2. Images of Dyslexia in Media

their own dyslexia, but creating awareness about America's number one learning disability. The hope is they serve as an antidote to what the activist David Perry suggests are the "norm": stories about any disability that contain "nothing real." The actual concern surrounding those kinds of stories is that "they distract us from the real needs of the disability community, including 'better policy, changing norms, and real conversations about key issues. Inspiration porn makes us feel that everything is going to be okay.'"

In many news stories, his research suggests, "disabled individuals are rendered passive. They rarely get to speak for themselves, to communicate how they feel, or to express their desires. Their lack of competence is presumed." He poses the question whether the person with the disability gets to speak for him or herself often, if ever, and concludes that "these are the questions journalists need to learn to ask. Unfortunately, as long as inspiration porn goes viral, there's no incentive for them to do so, and that's a pity. We all have the right to be agents of our own stories, rather than objects for someone else's emotional high."[19]

Starting with Fred Friendly and carrying through, generationally, with Gabrielle Emanuel, the journalists in this book help us answer at least some of the questions posed here, and others. Through their experiences, which while unique are also representative, we hope to explore how journalists can do better by being more genuine when reporting on dyslexia. Their authentic voices are not only needed, but vital, in fostering understanding of what we refer to as "the invisible disability." If they inspire while illuminating, that is our goal, especially for the young people with dyslexia who every day in America are told they can't, while they know they can.

Chapter 3

Fred W. Friendly

"I guess the fact that I couldn't read well, or get my math right, or spell made me all the more determined to succeed somehow."—Fred W. Friendly

Introduction

Fred W. Friendly was born in New York, but spent most of his childhood and adolescence in Rhode Island, where he began what would become a legendary broadcasting career at WEAN radio in Providence. Much has been written about Mr. Friendly—his partnership with Edward R. Murrow at CBS Radio and, later, at CBS Television, leading to seminal and historic programs like *Hear It Now* and *See It Now*. With Murrow, he has been credited by some scholars as the "inventor" of television news documentary. His long and distinguished career is well known, including his presidency of CBS News. He was a distinguished professor at the Columbia Graduate School of Journalism, and he has been credited with having the initial concept that led to the development of what is now PBS. What is less well known about Fred Friendly is that, like one of every five Americans, he was dyslexic, a learning disability that he didn't know he had until late in life.

"I remember my earliest school years…. I was color blind. I had a horrible time trying to learn to read. In first grade, I recall my teacher telling me to color the cow brown. I colored the cow GREEN. It looked brown to me—but I was labeled. And I began to think I was stupid."[1]

Stupid was only one label. Retarded. Dumb. Troublesome. These were among the other adjectives used to describe those with Fred Friendly's problem back then, long before society had put a name on it.

The boy who would one day interview generals and presidents, become the powerful head of America's premier news organization, and teach at one of our nation's most prestigious universities, was also

Chapter 3. Fred W. Friendly

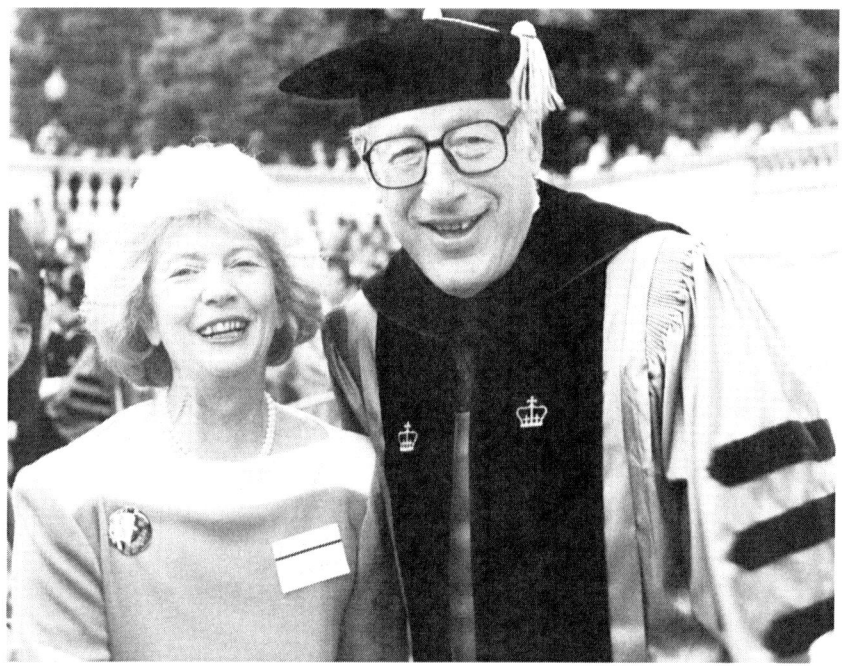

Ruth and Fred Friendly on the day that Fred received an honorary degree from Columbia University, 1986 (courtesy Ruth Friendly).

dyslexic. But few, even he, knew it at the time. In fact, it would be nearly five decades before he unraveled his own mystery.

His dream was right outside the window of his parents' home, but it might as well have existed in another solar system. The eleven-year-old made an imaginary microphone, using the round tubes from bathroom tissue. He taped them together so they looked like the real thing. He would then hold the "pretend" microphone up to his mouth and begin to speak. What came out was the description of what he saw, from outside his window and inside his mind. He pretended he was covering the news, on the air, as a reporter.[2]

"I could be a radio announcer," he thought to himself. "I could be on radio."

"He always said, 'I want to be a reporter,'" recalls one of the founders of the Hamilton School at Wheeler in Providence, Rhode Island, a place from which he would one day receive a Lifetime Achievement Award, the first ever bestowed by the school.

That was a long way off. Right then, in that moment, he had puzzles

Dyslexia and the Journalist

to solve in his head, puzzles that no one else around him, not his teachers, not his friends, not even his parents, could solve.

But that was his dream: to be a reporter, to "tell the news."

It was not an easy, possibly not even an achievable, dream for a boy with undiagnosed dyslexia, a condition for which there was no name at the time. He "had" something about which virtually *nothing* had been learned or discovered.

He wasn't alone, but he might as well have been. Dyslexia, at that time, was a kind of death sentence for a kid with dreams and intelligence, but also for whom reading and math were a challenge. And Fred Friendly was among them.

He was born Ferdinand Friendly Wachenheimer in New York in 1915 and moved to Rhode Island with his parents at age eleven. His father died of meningitis soon after the family moved to a home on Lloyd Avenue, on the east side of Providence. The young "Ferd," as he was then called by family and schoolmates, was big for his age, what some might describe as a "bear" of a young man. Because of that, he was somewhat of an awkward child, but his childhood difficulties extended far beyond the physical.

His mother, Therese Friendly Wachenheimer, was left on her own to raise a son who was "different" from the other boys his age. She was, by all accounts, a fierce advocate for young Fred, as he would eventually be called. A nurturing advocate for a son who was misunderstood by many teachers and other students, Therese had the means and the will to help him with myriad problems.

For one, he was color blind. For another, numbers were a headache for him and forming letters—let alone handwriting—challenged his fine motor skills, which were never very good. Worst of all, his innate curiosity about the world couldn't be satiated by reading—since reading, despite his love of knowledge, was at times torturous. It wasn't that he couldn't read; he could. Before moving to Rhode Island, he attended grades 1 through 6 at PS 165 in New York City. It was the place where, years later, he would credit his teacher, Margaret Forhan, with patiently and steadfastly teaching him to read.[3]

"I really didn't learn to read until fourth grade," he would recall later in life. "And that was probably because I had a very patient, caring teacher, Miss Forhan."

It also helped that, at home, his mother was an avid reader, a lifelong *New York Times* subscriber, and somewhat of a news junkie. Therese passed along her love of reading to young Fred, and he reaped

Chapter 3. Fred W. Friendly

the benefits. Even after he initially learned to read, "reading was still a problem for me," he remembered in 1995.

"And yet," he told the group of students at the Hamilton School in Providence, "I didn't think that I was DUMB. I thought that I was just as smart as lots of those other kids in my class. I just couldn't do many of the skills that were demanded of me. It wasn't easy, though, because I had the feeling that most people thought I wasn't bright at all—and sometimes I began to believe that myself."

While, Fred couldn't keep up with other students his age in reading and writing skills, he did display certain gifts related to history and geography. Like many dyslexics, he learned differently and absorbed "ideas" in ways that, to this day, educators can't always explain or accommodate.

Throughout his life, he would be described by others as a "big picture, big idea guy," one who could discern patterns in subjects that interested him, the aforementioned history and geography among them. Despite his learning difficulties, he had no problem learning all the states and their capitals, as well as internalizing five facts about each U.S. president.

History also fascinated him. In fact, it was his best subject in school; during the last two years of junior high school, "85" in history was his highest grade.[4] He was especially transfixed by the lives of famous leaders, politicians, artists, scientists—the common denominator being those who had distinguished themselves by achieving greatness of a specific kind, whatever that might be.

While at Hope Street High School in Providence, he was awarded the annual Athletic Cup for his athletic ability and vigor, while he was passed over for that year's History Cup, which was given to the student who excelled in studying history. The rule was one cup per student, and, throughout his life, Fred would remember wishing the history recognition had been his, rather than the athletic one, though he was also a big, strong kid and a fine athlete. His mother, Therese, would point with pride that during one summer at camp, he "won a prize for proficiency in track and field.... He was an avid baseball fan and an admirer of the great Jewish slugger Hank Greenberg."[5]

The truth was, like many dyslexics, he wasn't a great student. He tried hard, yes, but still he was not a great student. He was a better orator than a writer, better at recitation than reading. His grades weren't up to par, mostly C's, but still those who knew him well never doubted his intelligence.

Of what we now know as typical among some dyslexics, he was a

Dyslexia and the Journalist

"cut up" in class and socially awkward, and there were even suspicions he might be deaf—or worse. At one point, he even attended the Rhode Island School for the Deaf, based on his "slow" absorption of classroom learning.

Still, the young Fred had something others might misunderstand. He knew implicitly what his interests were and he knew exactly where to satisfy them: the Providence Public Library, a somewhat counterintuitive setting for a boy with dyslexia. He would hone his reading skills through his love of research. His favorite topics centered on history; he was captivated by the biographies of great men throughout the history of civilization.

His teachers didn't know it. His mother didn't know it. His friends couldn't have imagined it, but Ferdinand Wachenheimer was on the brink of becoming Fred Friendly, bolstered by the very thing that had held him back: reading.

And what he was reading would influence the course of his career in more ways than even he could have imagined. It was the beginning of a journey that would define his life. It started with a single idea, the genesis of which was time spent at the Providence Public Library. It grew out of his passion for history, combined with a talent for storytelling,

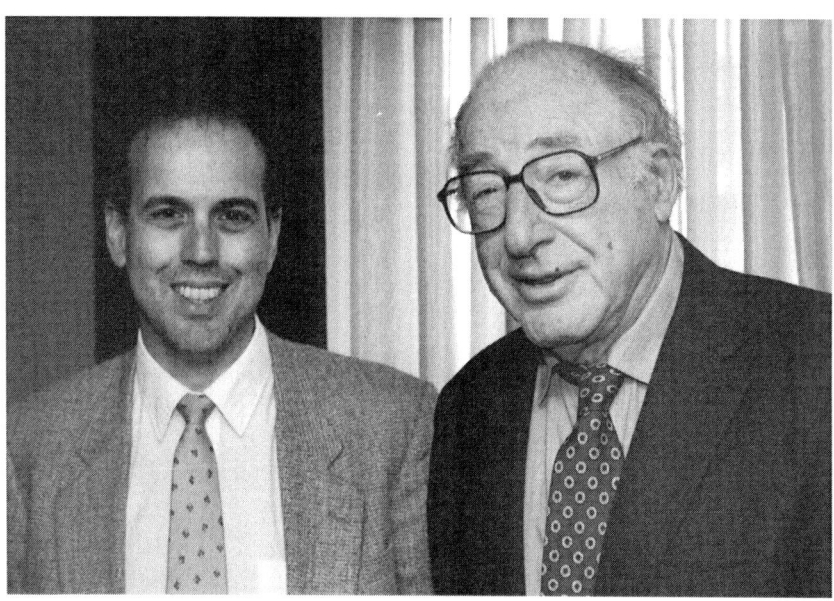

Fred Friendly (right) and Tony Silvia, at the University of Rhode Island, 1994.

Chapter 3. Fred W. Friendly

gained while acting in plays produced by a group of college women in Providence. They were always looking for men to play the male parts, and Fred happily participated.

The journey would eventually bring him to an actual microphone at a real radio station, to the war-torn capitals of Europe, to the christening of television, to the biggest stage of broadcast news, and, ultimately, to his own place in history.

Fred Friendly was nothing if not industrious. Today, the term entrepreneurial might aptly be used to describe him. After high school, he continued to live at home with his mother in a comfortable lifestyle; mother and son had a housekeeper and never struggled financially. Fred tried a variety of jobs: selling carpet in a department store, for one, and writing copy for an advertising agency, for another.

Still, the fire burned within him to achieve greater things, especially because others doubted his ability to do so. College had become an obsession. He had so much pride that, when other kids were applying to prestigious colleges, Fred touted the idea of going to Harvard, first to his high school guidance counselor and then to anyone who would listen.

The reality was that Nichols College, a small liberal arts school in Massachusetts, was the one school that would admit him, but even then, only after he attended a strict preparatory school program to improve his reading and study skills. Years later, he would formally and publicly recognize the role Nichols played in his success by taking a chance on a young man with undiagnosed dyslexia.

What no one, not even the youthful Fred himself, could have envisioned was that dyslexia, far from a curse, would actually become a blessing to someone in search of a childhood dream—in this instance, working in radio. The very skills his dyslexia brought him—determination, perseverance, impatience, attention to big ideas as opposed to minutiae, and a restless curiosity about those things that captured his imagination—would all be useful to a Providence radio station with the call letters WEAN.

According to Ruth Friendly, his widow, restlessness was a quality that served Fred Friendly well, especially in terms of the relatively new medium of radio. Ruth didn't meet her husband of thirty years until 1967, when he was fifty-two, but recalls how, even later in life, he was always trying to move, rearrange, or build things. "His mind was always going," she remembers. That applied not only to household activities but also to journalism, teaching, and business.

Fred was a thinker, some might say a visionary, who was always on the brink of innovation. His interest in radio may have been sparked when he was five years old. Radio was a relatively new medium at that time, and in its earliest days, radio receivers came in a box with parts that needed to be assembled. His father assembled the radio and gave it to Fred so the two could listen to one of the first prize fights ever broadcast. Ruth Friendly recalls her husband telling her his dad handed him one of the earpieces so they could listen to the boxing match together, transmitted from KDKA in Pittsburgh, one of America's seminal radio stations. The connection to radio stuck, as did the fascination with history and historical figures; the two became intertwined following his college graduation.

After college, Fred wrote to WEAN for over a year asking for work. At one point, he was asked in for a tour of the station and became fascinated with what, for its time, was new technology. He was dazzled by the idea of recording and radio's potential for storytelling. That same fascination stayed with him for life, yielding a love not only for radio, but also for learning new and different ways of looking at the world. Radio's major feature, audio, the spoken word, was perfect for a young man with dyslexia.

Fortuitously, James Jennison was WEAN's station manager at the time and took the young Fred under his wing. He recognized that Fred had "something," but just couldn't pinpoint what it was about him that made him stand out. Ultimately, Jennison would become one of Fred's earliest and most influential mentors. It was 1937 and the collaboration resulted in a series of programs titled *Footprints on the Sands of Time*.[6]

The name came from Fred's aunt (though the original source was a Longfellow poem) and *Footprints on the Sands of Time* consisted of five-minute biographies of prominent people and great historic figures.[7] Among those profiled were George Gershwin, Albert Einstein, Guglielmo Marconi (radio's inventor), the great conductor Arturo Toscanini, and Lou Gehrig. Each five-minute program brought Fred $15, welcome money at a time when it was very much needed.

He never gave up on the idea of that radio job in his adopted hometown of Providence. Of WEAN, he would say, "They were too big time for me—they thought. They told me to go north to Springfield and North Adams—but I ended up coming back to them—and I finally did get a job doing an idea that I had."[8]

Once he got that first break in radio, he could use his own natural interest in history to read what he needed to learn in order to produce the *Footprints* series. It was education by design—or necessity.

Chapter 3. Fred W. Friendly

"I could do five-minute biographies of great people and make it interesting. But how could I tell about these great men and women without doing research on them? WHAT SAVED ME??? THE PROVIDENCE PUBLIC LIBRARY," he would tell his audience many years in the future.[9] After college, it became his home away from home.

In addition to the *Footprints on the Sands of Time* vignettes, he took on announcer work, principally for a program titled *Streets of the City*, which was hosted by another WEAN staffer, Mowry Lowe. Eventually, he was promoted and continued his rise in Providence radio. He even became known as "Mr. Providence" on the radio, and his salary rose to $125 a week, a princely sum for someone who had struggled in school and appeared not to be chosen for success. Still, he was resourceful and ambitious. He really proved himself in covering the news during the historic hurricane of 1938 that caused massive, widespread damage across Rhode Island.

But the lasting mark from his early radio days was the aforementioned *Footprints on the Sands of Time* program. In it, he used his inordinate and refined audio skills, substituting verbal renditions of stories for written words. It was a palette on which he could freely paint without inhibition or self-consciousness, and he made the most of his strong oratorical sense. Ironically, his early learning disabilities also created in the young Fred the hint of a speech impediment, yet another challenge he had to overcome. Sound and speech were to become his refuge, the transformation of the words he struggled to read coming "alive" though a new medium that was uniquely suited to his specific talents.

Fred Friendly would describe himself as a "good talker." Words made sense when he heard them and he could make sense of them for others, he realized. "One thing I could do—I could speak well—and I had a good vocabulary," he once said. "I used to think and wonder about how I could ever earn a living." Radio was that breakthrough moment.

Not content to sit still, he continued to explore other ways to make money in the radio business, selling customized programs to local advertising agencies and producing radio shows for clients of all kinds. By this time, he was known as Fred W. Friendly (he reversed his surname with his mother's maiden name to create the middle initial "W"). The catalyst was that same station manager who had hired him at WEAN. In Fred's own words years later, "The manager said as he hired me, 'What did you say your name was?' I told him, and he said, 'Nobody on this station is named Wachenheimer. From now on, you're Fred W. Friendly!'"

Fred W. Friendly was well on his way to what would become a

Dyslexia and the Journalist

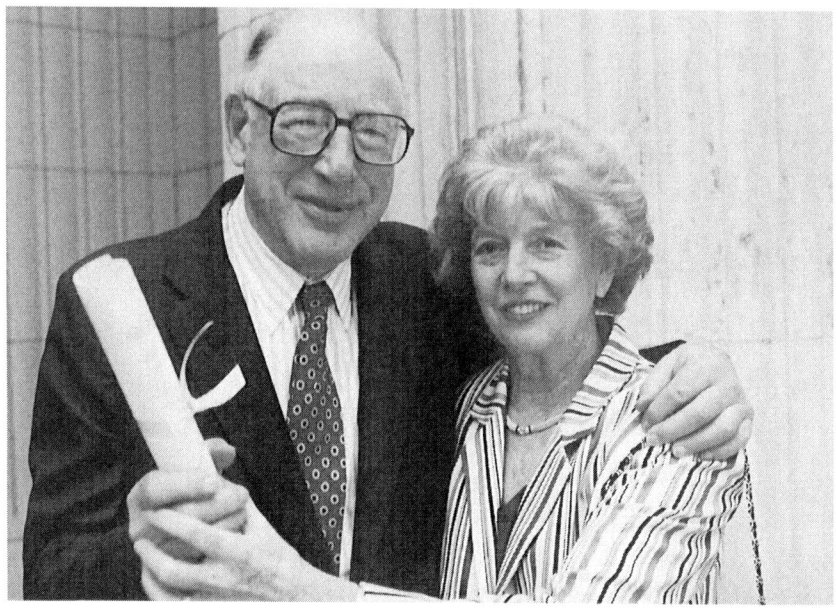

Fred and Ruth Friendly at Quinnipiac University in 1994 (courtesy Ruth Friendly).

legendary career in broadcasting, but not before he—and thousands of other young men—were forced to put their dreams on hold. The reason was World War II. For rising radio star Fred W. Friendly, it could have been a setback, but instead the war brought new opportunities that he couldn't have envisioned, but of which he certainly took full advantage.

In 1941, the newly named Fred W. Friendly, "Mr. Providence," found himself in the U.S. Army on KP duty, a humbling experience. His first assignment, after being drafted, was kitchen duty. His job was to put sliced onions on liver and onion dinners for 1,500 soldiers. He hated the scent of liver and onions, so it was not a job for which he was well suited; nor was it how he wanted to leave his mark on the war.[10]

Soon, he would find ways to convince his superior officers that he had more to offer. He convinced those in command he could use his voice to inspire and instruct soldiers in their combat missions. In other words, he became, in his own way, a "teacher," once addressing 10,000 troops in a motivational speech. From there on, he had a new role, driving from camp to camp, using his powerful voice to instruct the troops.

"Believe it or not, I became a teacher of thousands and thousands of men," he would relate years later. "I could hardly believe it. Little did

Chapter 3. Fred W. Friendly

I dream that one day I would be working with General Eisenhower and General Stillwell." One army major, whom the young soldier considered a role model, thought so highly of Friendly that he considered him worthy of receiving the Legion of Merit for his efforts in raising morale.

"How could this be happening to me—the dope in school," Friendly asked himself. Major Clark wrote, "Fred Friendly, in my estimation, has made the most significant and outstanding contribution to the Information and Education of any enlisted man in the Army today. Many of his unique [teaching] techniques have been adopted by other commands."

By this time, Friendly was also working his way back into radio, at least the army's version of radio. He began by doing reporting of the kind he'd developed while at WEAN, recording the sounds of combat, interviewing soldiers, and creating compelling story lines that would be heard by both the troops and those back home in the United States.

He used the recording standard of the day—a wire recorder—to go up in planes and capture the actual sounds of the war. Ruth Friendly recalls how, in later years, Fred would love to tell the story of how he would do the recordings by trying to splice the wires together using a lit cigarette butt while on the fighter plane—a practice that made others on the plane wince in fear that it would blow up. There's another account of how Fred did a report from the bedside of an injured combat pilot undergoing surgery. He "held the sterilized microphone an inch from the knife as it cut the man's abdomen. The reports captured the words of the patient, the nurses, and the surgeon, who, at the end despaired of saving the patient."[11]

The accolades for Fred Friendly began to mount. "His radio reporting, his development of the Orientation Quiz program, his project for shipboard orientation, are only a few of the many procedures which have made the mission in this theater far easier," wrote Major Clark, his commanding officer, when praising Friendly's accomplishments. "But even beyond these things, Friendly will have made his greatest contribution in his inspired ability to stand before a group of American soldiers and tell a simple, yet eloquent and important story, which will leave a profound influence for good in the lives of those who have him."[12]

The young Fred Friendly's achievements not only surprised others; they also baffled him. Reflecting back to those days toward the end of his life, he would tell an audience of students, "Could that really be the same Fred Friendly who couldn't learn to read for so long, whose spelling was atrocious, whose math seemed beyond repair?"[13]

It was and it wasn't. Still not sure of what it was that had threatened

Dyslexia and the Journalist

to hold him back, he had found a way to move forward, partly out of perseverance, mostly out of the will arising from a phrase he adopted from the writer E. B. White who used the term "willing to be lucky." And his next stroke of luck was just around the corner.

Luck came in the form of those five-minute vignettes that added up to a library of almost a thousand biographies: *Footprints on the Sands of Time*, which had begun life as a radio feature during his four years at Providence's WEAN (1937–41). Sound was evolving from radio to records that people could play in their homes. For Fred Friendly to become a part of that movement, he needed two things—three, really—encouragement, support, and, yes, luck.

There was a lot of good fortune that occurred during this time. While at Camp Koler, Major Clark allowed him the time to continue recording his *Footprints* programs for WEAN and send them back to Providence. It wasn't his initial idea to put the *Footprints* programs on records. That came from Jack Kapp, then founder and head of Decca Records. While still in the army, Fred received a call from Kapp offering him $25,000 for the series.

Once the war ended, in 1947, a second stroke of good luck came Fred Friendly's way. He was introduced to Edward R. Murrow, then CBS Radio's biggest star. Murrow had covered the war in Europe as a soothing, familiar voice to Americans glued to their radio sets each evening awaiting news from the battlefields and rooftops. Murrow was six years Friendly's senior and a major radio presence, for reasons stated. He had credibility, clout, and charisma.

The two—Friendly and Murrow—were introduced in 1947 by their mutual agent, J. G. (nicknamed Jap) Gude. The meeting led to a collaboration that resulted in *Hear It Now*, first on CBS Radio and then as a collection of records. One remarkable part of the series is that the original voices of the historical figures profiled were featured on the recordings. Here again, Fred Friendly was a visionary. He saw how technology was changing the landscape for, among other things, disseminating news. "America now has a bottomless appetite for news," he once stated, and he "emphasized the unrealized potential of recordings to bring to radio the voices of the world and to create a permanent record of those sounds."[14]

Decca, which had released his *Footprints* on record, turned down *Hear It Now*, but Columbia Records signed a deal with Murrow and Friendly to release the recordings. Ruth Friendly remembers how excited her husband was to have audio tape—as opposed to the old

Chapter 3. Fred W. Friendly

wire recordings used during the war—to make the *Hear It Now* records. "As Fred put it to me, when audio tape became available, he realized he could do clean edits of the speeches of famous people, which gave birth to the idea of *Hear It Now*."[15]

With Murrow, Friendly would go on not only to produce some of the most seminal radio news documentaries, but also, utilizing the power, prominence, and stature of Murrow, to help invent the use of television as a news medium.[16] While Murrow would gain a place in history as "the father of broadcast news," many scholars agree that it was Friendly who pushed him toward the upstart medium of television as a purveyor of news and information for mass audiences.

The result was the transfer of *Hear It Now* on radio to *See It Now* on television. This included several historic programs, conceived and written by both Murrow and Friendly, including the most famous one involving Senator Joseph McCarthy's communist "witch hunt."[17] It was a program that utilized the power of TV for what Friendly throughout his life thought it should be: the education and elucidation of Americans on important public policy issues.

Fred Friendly functioned throughout those years as an undiagnosed dyslexic, achieving at the highest levels of radio and television, without acknowledging those factors in his childhood that might have held him back. If anything, his widow, Ruth Friendly, asserts, it drove him forward. Then came a day in 1974 when the light bulb went on, and his family, friends, and Fred himself could put a name to what had challenged him for the previous sixty years.

Ruth Friendly recalls the day in 1974 when she came home from teaching fifth grade at the Heathcote School in New York. It had been an enlightening day, involving one student in particular. She relayed the challenges she was facing with this bright boy who was very verbal, smart, and capable, but who wasn't reading or spelling well and had writing issues. "I told Fred that I had the idea of letting the student record his report on a tape recorder and that worked very well because he spoke very well." After hearing of her challenges with this student, Fred had an epiphany that these signs and symptoms were exactly what his struggles had been ... and he recognized that he, too, was dyslexic. As he remembered of that day, "She was describing ME in elementary school. That is when I became interested in people who had the same learning difficulties that I did. So many of them found ways to get around their problems."[18]

It was an "aha" moment, one that, in some ways, was as much a surprise to his family as it was to him. As Fred's second wife, Ruth hadn't known him during his youthful days in Providence when dyslexia most challenged him and asserts to this day that it never held him back (as evidenced by his amazing accomplishments). There were signs, but none of them, by his fifties, had to do with reading; math, however, continued to plague him. As late as 1995, he admitted to an audience of listeners, "I don't think that I could pass a math test, honestly—even now."[19]

Another challenge throughout his life was handwriting. Ruth Friendly remembers how his handwriting was bad due to his fine motor skills and computers weren't a good alternative. He would hit the keys so hard that the same letter would repeat over and over. Never daunted, in his later life, Fred wrote four books, all in CAPS using the "hunt and peck method" on a typewriter. He would also write hundreds of speeches in longhand. And he never stopped reading, before, during, or after recognizing his dyslexia.

His daughter, Lisa Friendly, had always heard as a child that her father struggled with dyslexia, but never saw evidence of it in the Friendly household:

> I heard all about that ... but to me, he had become such an intellectual. He was so smart and was the smartest person that most of us knew, that my friends knew, and so I always felt that your mind tries to put this together and I always felt that dyslexia is either something that you outgrow or overcome, because my dad was this brilliant intellectual who showed no signs of difficulty reading. I remember that he was always reading these very thick books. He had a reading chair in his den and was always reading about civil rights and current affairs, and whatever new book was out. It was ironic to me, although I didn't use that word ironic when I was young, but he was such a towering intellectual and I think he read more than most parents you know. So, he had this incredible love of words.[20]

She described the family home being filled with books and a nightly dinner table ritual, where their father would quiz Lisa and her brothers on current events, politics, history, and philosophy: all areas in which he expected them to be knowledgeable and conversant. He also encouraged them to read books that challenged them, not necessarily ones that were popular at the time and to take on complex topics about which to write. "When I had to write a biography in high school, he suggested ... forcefully ... no enthusiastically ... that what I write about was the conflict between Disraeli and Gladstone for the election in England of prime minister, in which I had no intrinsic interest. But I did that and ended up reading all of these books and he was just like, 'THIS is what you gotta

Chapter 3. Fred W. Friendly

do!' So, I became this big reader. I love words, write well, spell very well, and it has passed right on to my children who also love reading books."

The man and father who had to work arduously at reading wanted his children to recognize and appreciate the gift they possessed naturally. And his efforts weren't solely centered on books. "He went through a phase where we had to bring in articles from the newspaper to the dinner table and explain what they were about," Lisa Friendly remembers. "That lasted a couple of years. Yeah, it was just this—You will be aware of current affairs. I felt that was the thing that distinguished him the most, as the most intellectual dad amongst my friends."

What also distinguished Fred Friendly—and is common to what we now know of dyslexics—is the fervor with which he would approach problems, always searching for new ideas and solutions. Ruth Friendly would observe that he found it difficult to "leave things as they are," preferring instead innovation—whether it was in broadcasting or teaching or myriad other areas that interested him. People said of Fred that he had one hundred new ideas a day, only four of which were good. Fred would tell his assistants and those who worked under his leadership in jest, "it's your job to find those four."

That drive toward the "big ideas" began in the books read by a restless college graduate back in the Providence Public Library, and they paid Fred Friendly major dividends throughout his life. In 1964, on the heels of award-winning documentaries done with Murrow on *CBS Reports* on topics like the exploitation of migrant farm workers ("Harvest of Shame") and, of course, the 1954 McCarthy *See It Now* broadcast, Fred Friendly ascended to the highest position at CBS News, that of president, a position he held until 1966.

After leaving CBS, he assumed the Edward R. Murrow Professorship at the esteemed Columbia Graduate School of Journalism in 1966. Among other accomplishments there, he headed its broadcast journalism division and founded a mentoring program for minority journalists. He simultaneously worked with the Ford Foundation. He would leave Columbia in the afternoon to go across town and work on another of his passions, an educational role for television. In 1967, his vision for television as a public service involved the origination of public access TV cable channels—the forerunner of today's PBS. Together with a team and Ruth Friendly as a key player, he produced an influential series of media seminars on timely issues. There were over five hundred seminars, of which eighty odd were broadcast on PBS.[21]

Perhaps most importantly is that once he recognized his learning disability had a name—dyslexia—he never shied away from or hid from it. If anything, Ruth Friendly says, he "advertised his dyslexia." In that 1995 speech at Providence's Hamilton School, Fred Friendly brought recognition to another high-achieving dyslexic. "Today, many people are aware of the problems some of us have," he began. "Just the other day there was a story about a famous scientist in California, Dr. Don Francis. He is working on a vaccine for the disease AIDS." In addition, Friendly pointed out, "he has already helped to eradicate other terrible illnesses all over the world. Imagine my surprise as I read Francis had grown up in San Francisco, the DYSLEXIC HIPPY CHILD OF TWO DOCTORS."[22]

He was fascinated both by the irony and the majesty of the achievement. "He found a way, probably with help from understanding teachers, to get around those problems, probably similar to the ones that plagued me for so many years. He is being taken seriously all over the world today and he is dyslexic."

In his later years, Fred Friendly's desire to be taken seriously became part of the drive that led him to be as tough on his students and his own kids as he was on himself. "There are always some things that are hard for a person to do. Some people can't run fast, or swim well, or draw beautifully, or dance, or sing. I guess the fact that I couldn't read well, or get my math right, or spell made me all the more determined to succeed somehow."[23]

Fred Friendly's contributions—to broadcasting, to education, to history, and to government—can be considered stellar in any context, but they shine even brighter against the dark sky that some experience as dyslexia. "Somewhere, in spite of all that trouble, some people helped me develop faith in myself," were his final words in that 1995 speech focusing on the challenges and victories of those with dyslexia. Within those words lies a challenge: Have faith in those who are different, so they can build faith in themselves.

Chapter 4

Anderson Cooper

"School can be an incredibly isolating place. It can be a place that's frustrating and, frankly, overwhelming."—Anderson Cooper

Since 2003, Anderson Cooper has been the primary anchor on CNN's *Anderson Cooper 360*. He also has been a correspondent for CBS's *60 Minutes* and previously worked in various on-air capacities at ABC News.

Where Fred Friendly is considered to be one of the most formative TV journalists of his time, CNN's Anderson Cooper may be considered among the most influential of his time.[1] There are those who might even consider Cooper a close descendant of Fred Friendly, at least in terms of broadcast news. For one, his experience has spanned the globe, much as Friendly's did, in his early journalism years. For another, he has made a career of "keeping them honest," a mantra he embraces nightly on his CNN broadcast *Anderson Cooper 360*.[2] That is, of course, exactly what Fred Friendly and Edward R. Murrow did when holding politicians' and demagogues' feet to the fire during their legendary *See It Now* programs on CBS.

And, though two generations removed from Fred Friendly, the two also share another thing in common: dyslexia. There is a major difference, however. While Fred Friendly spent most of his youth not knowing he was dyslexic, Anderson Cooper always knew, from an early age. The signs were there. The diagnosis was present. The resources existed. None of the above was true for Fred Friendly or others of his generation.

"When I was a kid, I was diagnosed with a mild form of dyslexia," Cooper told a luncheon audience at the National Center for Learning Disabilities in 2010. He discussed how his older brother was a very good reader, so Anderson would also carry a book around with him. The idea was to make it appear to others that he, too, could read. "But I was never actually reading the book. I would just pretend to read because I couldn't make sense of the words and, in particular, letters."³

Fortunately, his parents had both the resources and the will to send him to a private elementary school. It was there where the problem was first recognized and diagnosed. "Luckily, I went to a school that caught the problem very quickly and diagnosed it. I had access to people who could really help."

The next step was sending him to a reading specialist: "I remember a couple of times a week I would go to a doctor named Dr. Jansky, who I called my reading doctor. I really didn't know what she was."

"I remember at the time, I was concerned that other people would find out about it and I didn't want the kids in my class to find out about it because I went to this special place. At the time, I think part of the treatment was learning how to type. I'm not sure exactly why, but I'm quite a good typer now, so I thank her for that," he said with a laugh, when addressing the luncheon audience.

As a result, Anderson Cooper has become insistent that early intervention is crucial. "To me, it's just a sign of the importance a school plays in a child's life and in particular a child with a learning disability," he adds. "To a child with learning disabilities, school can be an incredibly isolating place. It can be a place that's frustrating and, frankly, overwhelming. It's vital that kids have access to teachers who can meet their unique needs. Too many kids with learning disabilities struggle to keep up with their peers and suffer from low confidence and self-esteem."

In fact, studies show a direct relationship between dyslexia and low self-confidence.⁴ There are a variety of reasons, most of them intuitive. Part of the problem is they don't have a stress-free, nonjudgmental environment in which to practice their reading skills. Most also aren't provided with incentives to tackle or improve their reading. Finally, they and their parents don't know where to turn for help, either in the community, online, or through social media. That reinforces a sense of isolation that feeds low self-confidence. As Cooper sees it, "they lose their love of learning and it's hard to rekindle that once it's gone."

In his speech to the National Center for Learning Disabilities, Cooper showed awareness of the studies supporting the idea that students with any learning disability "are retained in grade much more often than other students, and they're involved in school disciplinary actions in far greater numbers and at a much higher rate than their nondisabled peers." Nearly a quarter of all students with learning disabilities drop out of high school, he pointed out, and "only about 60 percent actually earn a high school diploma, so not all students are getting what they need to find success in school."

Elementary school, he says, makes "all the difference. It made all the difference in my life early on." He sees hope because "the good news that we know is that there are good schools out there that are able to provide the necessary resources and support for students with learning disabilities. The majority of our nation's schools, though, are not up to the challenge," he continued during the same address.

His own dyslexia, self-characterized as "mild," aside, in some ways Anderson Cooper had reading and writing in his genes. His father was Wyatt Emory Cooper, a writer who also sometimes dabbled in acting. According to one account, he always admired his father's ability to write, as well as the sound of his keyboard. It probably also helped that, on his mother's side, he was exposed at an early age to a range of highly artistic, literate, and visually oriented people: in other words, writers and those in the movie industry. His mother, Gloria Vanderbilt, of the famous Vanderbilt clan, gave him the pedigree of one of America's wealthiest families.[5]

Because his parents led a prominent social life, the young Anderson was able to party with people like the actress Lillian Gish, the journalist George Plimpton, and even the legendary Charlie Chaplin. He moved in all the right circles because he had that level of access. Yet, from an early age, as one account put it, despite the privilege that came with his heritage, "he would work his way to prominence the old-fashioned way, through grit and perseverance, and he'd overcome various obstacles along the way, some life threatening, and some downright outrageous."[6]

Cooper was fortunate in that regard. The son of heiress Gloria Vanderbilt, he found resources more readily available than for other kids with dyslexia. His parents also encouraged him not just to carry a book around with him, but to read books. "Eventually, I read *Heart of Darkness*," he once said in an interview of the novel by British author Joseph Conrad. "That novel, in particular, sparked an interest in seeing what happens in society when everything is stripped away, when you're living without the niceties of modern culture."

It was his mother's idea, initially, to have a home surrounded in books. "Some people grow up in homes where sports are important; I grew up in a home where reading and writing had great value." He gives credit also to the special reading instructor to whom his parents sent him. "One way she helped was to encourage me to find books that I was really passionate about." In addition to his affinity for *Heart of Darkness*,

Dyslexia and the Journalist

Cooper also came to love the story of Helen Keller. He read her biography and saw similarities at any early age between it and Conrad's *Heart of Darkness*: it was the common theme of survival.[7]

"I don't think it's an accident that I became a war correspondent," he said in an interview. "I'm interested in stories of survival: how some people make it through desperate times and others don't. If you go to a conflict zone, you find there's never a complete vacuum. There's always some form of authority. It may not make sense, and it's terrifying. You learn that people are capable of horrific brutality but also great kindness. You see things straight out of Conrad—and how a novel from the 1890s still resonates today."[8]

He didn't stop with Conrad and Keller. Once reading captured Anderson Cooper's imagination, he moved on to other writers who held a special significance, the author James Agee being one of them, specifically the novel *A Death in the Family*. "This is about what happens after the unexpected death of a father. Certainly, the novel had resonance for me because I lost my father at an early age and this book is told from the vantage point of the young son," he recalled. Cooper's father died when he was ten, and his brother committed suicide when he was in early adulthood.

"Dealing with grief is difficult, especially for a child. There are peaks and valleys—grief has a life of its own—and Agee does a good job of exploring that territory. The book opens with a scene of people—men with wives and children—watering their lawns while cicadas are buzzing. There's a poetry to the writing in that it describes events that really cannot be described." His fascination with grief and survival began to take many forms.

While attending the private university preparatory Dalton School in Manhattan, he was exposed not only to strong academics, but also the arts. His thirst for reading accelerated. It also gained a focus leading him take a course in, of all things, human survival. It fed his curiosity and ultimately led to explorations outside the classroom, with trips to the Rocky Mountains and Mexico. But his curiosity about far-off places didn't end there.

After graduating high school a semester early, Cooper decided to explore the globe more broadly. He decided to go out into the wilderness to study survival up close. That first took him to Africa. He was seventeen when he decided to go backpacking on his own through Central Africa. According to one account of his travels, plans went awry. He ended up with malaria, spending time hospitalized in Kenya. At that

Chapter 4. Anderson Cooper

point, adventures in survival closer to home seemed a better idea, so, once cured, he returned to the United States and set his sights on college. Ultimately, he ended up studying political science at Yale, but he remained uncertain of a career path.

As will often happen, an unexpected turn created clarity, if not opportunity. He saw a flyer in the university's career counseling office that proved fortuitous. It advertised an opportunity for students to try out the CIA—yes, that CIA, the Central Intelligence Agency—as a summer experience. He signed up and, ultimately, ended up spending two summers interning with the CIA. It wasn't all he envisioned: too "bureaucratic" and "mundane," he recalled.

He was close to graduation when tragedy struck. That's when his brother took his own life. It brought back to Anderson Cooper the whole idea of survival, in a very personal way. He began to ask himself, as he put it, "why some people survive and others don't."[9] Through suffering and serendipity, that question—and its accompanying curiosity coupled with pain—brought him to journalism.

According to one account, it's what ultimately led him to become a war correspondent. "Covering wars just seemed logical," he once said.[10] There was a small problem. He had no reporting experience, and he had never covered a war. Still, he had a political science degree and a desire to travel, so how hard could it be? He found out quickly that the world wasn't waiting for Anderson Cooper, so he had to make his own opportunity. After not getting a job after applying at ABC, he decided to freelance as a war correspondent, which meant he didn't have a job and no salary beyond the stories he could sell to any news organization that was willing to pay.

Early on, his parents made it clear to both sons that, despite their enormous Vanderbilt wealth, they would receive no inheritance. They would have to make it on their own. It came as no shock to Cooper that he would have to find his own way.[11] Then again, one of the lessons of having dyslexia is exactly that: finding your own way, sometimes with the help of others, but often not.

To get into journalism, he bought his own camera, forged press passes, and fronted his own way to war zones around the globe, beginning with Burma and Somalia. He shot his own stories, did his own interviews, and somehow crafted stories, despite having zero reporting experience. In some ways, that was the easy part; gaining an audience for his work was far more difficult.

Fortunately, his timing was right. A classroom-based television network named Channel One had recently started up. Its owners were impressed with Cooper's tenacity, his willingness to go where other reporters wouldn't. Focused on media literacy, Channel One had a national audience ranging from elementary to high school students. It began in 1990 and folded in 2018, but, in its earliest days, it was a great start for the young Anderson Cooper. He was named a full-time correspondent, a job that took him around the globe. And it created other advantages.

For one, the network allowed him to pack up and spend time in Vietnam, learn Vietnamese, study at the University of Hanoi, and produce stories about his experiences that Channel One would broadcast back in America. He was learning, both about journalism and a different country—and getting paid to do both. It was almost like getting a graduate school education for free, which, for a kid who had struggled with mild dyslexia in his youth, was not lost on Anderson Cooper or on those who knew him.

For another, he was noticed by other mainstream broadcast and cable networks, among them ABC, where he had once been rejected for an entry-level job. The ABC brass was impressed with the reporting credentials he had gained while at Chanel One, especially the self-made nature of his success.[12] They gave him a number of assignments, reporting on all their platforms, from the flagship *ABC World News Tonight* to anchoring its overnight *World News Now* broadcast.

He eventually became one of the youngest war correspondents in the network's history. In his memoir, *Dispatches from the Edge: A Memoir of War, Disasters, and Survival* (2007), he recalled how the fast-paced life of a war correspondent, constantly travelling, facing deadlines, danger, and even potential death, helped him avoid his own personal pain and grief for a long time. From the tsunami in Sri Lanka to the Iraq War, genocide in Rwanda, and, closer to home, Hurricane Katrina, it was a far cry and a major leap from the comfortable Upper East Side life into which he was born.[13]

Cooper kept moving, whether from avoidance of personal pain or ambition (or perhaps both), and so did his career.

In 2001, he switched from ABC to CNN, where, since 2003, he has anchored his own prime-time news program, *Anderson Cooper 360*. Through a cooperative agreement, he was also allowed to be a contributor to rival network CBS's legacy news magazine, *60 Minutes*. Throughout a career that has included winning every prestigious journalism award and reporting on topics from politics to corruption, and moderating presidential debates, Cooper has stood firm as a strong advocate for improving both understanding of and resources for those with dyslexia.

Like others in this book, he says there are still those who are surprised when they discover he has dyslexia. Even those who have known him for a long time, both coworkers and friends, find it hard to believe, given his many accomplishments and accolades. He attributes that, in part, to how well he concealed his learning disability as a child, something that, as we have discussed, is not at all unusual in children with dyslexia—or their parents. "I think it's a sign of probably how well I tried to hide it when I was a little kid. I remember at the time being concerned that other people would find out about it."[14]

To this day, while he no longer hides it, his dyslexia is not readily apparent to those in his circle of coworkers. At least two high-profile CNN colleagues with whom we spoke admitted that they had no idea he is dyslexic. That's despite the fact that he has written and spoken on the topic publicly on many occasions and has never shied away from it when it's addressed in interviews. He doesn't make it a part of who he is, but instead as a vehicle to show how far he has come and, by extension, how far others with dyslexia, or any form of learning disability, can go.

In terms of learning and having goals, he has been quoted as saying "learning what you don't want to do is the next best thing to learning what you want to do." More importantly, perhaps, is the idea of coming out of the shadows and into the light. As with many dyslexics or others with learning disabilities, visibility is the key to change or, as Anderson Cooper puts it, "the tide of history only advances when people make themselves fully visible."[15]

Chapter 5

Byron Pitts

> "The school sent my mom and me to an outside evaluator and their response was that I was mentally retarded."— Byron Pitts

Byron Pitts has spent a distinguished career in television news, first with CBS News, where he served as chief national correspondent for *The CBS Evening News*, as well as reporting for its signature news magazine, *60 Minutes*. In 2013, he moved to ABC News, where he currently is the co-anchor for the late-night news program *Nightline*.

Twelve-year-old Byron Pitts knew he was different. So did his mother and his siblings. Good athletically, he was challenged in just about every other area of his life at school.

"I played football primarily and wrestled through college. Sports were very important to me and I was active in my church, so sports and singing in the church choir helped sustain me," he recalls.[1]

He started in public school, but soon his reading and writing problems overtook him and, out of care and somewhat desperation, his mom, Clarice, looked for other options to help her son. "My mother put me in Catholic school in elementary school and I went to an all-boys Catholic high school, in part because of my academic issues. And certainly, by the time I was 9 or 10, there were issues of self-esteem because I was very aware that I was different from other kids."

It didn't help that he had, by that age, developed a severe stuttering problem and his reading had become so bad that he now recognizes himself as having been functionally illiterate. Raised by a single mother, Pitts endured teasing by classmates, derision by teachers, and the kind of social ostracism that often accompanies the kid who can't read, the "dummy," the "lazy ass," the kid who no one knew and who no one wanted to get to know. Byron Pitts had become the invisible kid.

At least life at home was better. "No teasing was done at all to me by my siblings, and my mother was insistent that we be our best friends,

Chapter 5. Byron Pitts

confidants, and supporters. So there was no teasing ... my older brother and sister were fully supportive." That was fortunate because life at school was hardly nurturing. "I was bullied through elementary school and much of junior high school.... I didn't have many friends because of my stutter. I was embarrassed a lot of times and out of that embarrassment came anger and isolation."

In fact, his older brother was, in many ways, a mentor and a willing accomplice—someone who helped with his trouble reading, while at the same time assisting him in hiding what he now says was functional illiteracy. In an interview with NPR, he recalled convincing his older brother to read out loud from one of his school books at night and then memorizing all the words in a single paragraph for the next day's class.

When the teacher got to that paragraph, he'd volunteer to read. "I had it down to a science," he recalls. "I would raise my hand, actually, two or three sentences before I got to the graph Id memorized to let the teacher know I was interested. And, in fact, if she called on me before we got to the sentence I memorized, I would say, oh, no. That's okay. Let Johnny read it."[2]

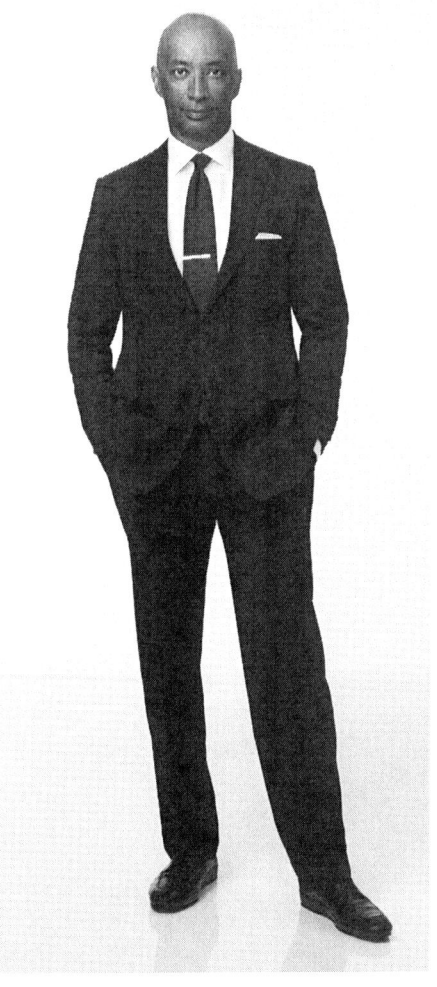

Byron Pitts, co-anchor of *Nightline* (courtesy ABC News).

That strategy worked for *and* against him. "Children learn to read from birth to seven, and from seven on they read to learn," he says. "Somewhere in those early years, I just missed the basics. I didn't learn

Dyslexia and the Journalist

to read. Because of my speech problems, I was quiet in general. But I was well-mannered and somehow it was assumed I knew the material well enough to keep me passing from grade to grade."

His illiteracy was discovered, ironically, not through a failure to read out loud, but when Pitts was in the sixth grade and failed math because he couldn't read the questions or directions. Next came a remedial program, but there were still spurts and starts to his learning. Eventually, he saw an advertisement for a remedial reading program and his mother, who had worked hard to attain her own GED, devised the means to give her son access.

Thanks to the remedial reading program, he made significant strides toward literacy, not full, but at least strides. He was able to return to his regular school classes. To reinforce his reading, his mother began leaving him notes containing Bible quotes each morning. "I loved getting those notes," he says, adding that they provided a positive, optimistic approach, the idea that he could and would get there. He would read. He would succeed. It's probably not coincidental that his mother's favorite book was *The Power of Positive Thinking* by Norman Vincent Peale.

To this day, he calls himself a "visual learner," not an uncommon characteristic of those with dyslexia, and that wasn't his only advantage. "Well, I was blessed with a good memory. I could memorize things. I'm a picture reader, so I could recognize words and their context, and basically faked it. You know, according to the National Center for Family Literacy, there are 30 million adults in our country who are functionally illiterate, who can't read. That's one in seven adults in the most powerful country on earth. So, I wasn't alone."[3]

He might have been far from alone, in terms of his reading problems, but very much alone in solitary confinement in terms of social interaction. Between his stutter and his burgeoning reading difficulties, he was near crisis stage—and still far from his teenage years. "From my childish perspective, I was simply a freak: the strange one, the one who couldn't get the words out, couldn't do a simple thing like speak clearly. For me, it was like living as a prisoner inside a cell ... and the times I just wanted lemonade in the school cafeteria but could only say the word soda. I've never liked soda. Would never drink it if I had the choice.... At the time self-esteem was a term with little meaning in the world of a child, but it's clear to me now I had very little self-esteem back then."[4]

Then came the day when he was ten. The public schools weren't equipped to handle a kid like him, but they did recommend to his mother that he see an expert to figure out what could be done to help

Chapter 5. Byron Pitts

ease the stuttering and fight the illiteracy. His mother, a working-class woman with a tenth grade education that worked two jobs, was no expert, but she knew what her son needed.

Imagine. You're ten years old, and you're in the room, present and listening as you hear the "expert" give his verdict on what's plaguing you. It's not that you stutter or can't read. It's worse. "The opinion was that I was mentally retarded. Their words, not mine. So, the recommendation to my mother was that she institutionalize me. Because they thought there was no hope for me to lead, in their words, a normal life."

Not dyslexic. Not a learning disability. Not treatable or curable. The expert opinion was mental retardation and the recommendation was to put this ten-year-old kid in an institution, possibly for life. Fortunately, his mother didn't listen. In fact, she rebelled. In many ways, *she* became the expert in her own son's path and treatment.

Even then, the young Byron was motivated to succeed, mainly motivated by not wanting to see his mother in pain. "It was the first time I ever saw my mother cry. The moment was devastating. In fact, it was that moment that forged my own commitment to learn to read. To this point, I was resigned to be 'slow' and 'stupid,' as many classmates and a few adults referred to me at that stage of my life. In the beginning, I simply wanted to read so my mother wouldn't cry."[5]

Clarice Pitts was his role model, his safety blanket, his comfort, and his inspiration. As with many high-achieving dyslexics, Pitts's mom was his earliest and perhaps most important advocate, a common occurrence among so many dyslexic children. "My mother, she is passed away now, but my mother was a woman who believed there was nothing that hard work, prayer and optimism couldn't overcome." All three not only became her son's mantra, but also the path to a journey beyond dyslexia and into a life full of words, both spoken and written. It began with the stuttering, but the progression was eventually the diagnosis of dyslexia.

It's not unusual, in fact, it's fairly typical, for young people with dyslexia to also have a stuttering problem—and that was true for Pitts. Whether the two were related, his parents' divorce when he was twelve amplified the stuttering that had, up to that point, always been an issue. It also was in the DNA. "My father wasn't an active participant prior to that, but both of my parents had a stammer. So, there was this assumption, and because I was shy and had other issues going on I didn't talk much. So when I did, it was just like, well he has a stammer like the rest of us. But as I got older, it didn't get better and then I became more self-conscious about that. Then it got to the point where my siblings,

Dyslexia and the Journalist

and certainly my mother, would finish my sentences, in their efforts to protect and guard me ... you know my world was small, I didn't have a lot of friends outside of my immediate family."

Social isolation was another aspect of dyslexia that the young Byron Pitts both experienced and endured. It's a common thread, but, fortunately, he found refuge in spaces outside the home. "My activities were focused on church activities, my church community and sports. And neither one of those things required me to talk much. I could sing without talking. In fact, in many ways singing was easier for me than to talk. And then in playing sports, giving out a cadence, because I played quarterback and I was a team captain. So, there's sort of a cadence to that language. It can also be kind of like a song, the way you had to call out plays in a rhythmic fashion, so I could function in that space as well."

There were teachers who recognized his innate ability in certain areas, but not early on. "Certainly not in elementary school or high school," he remembers. "Certainly I did have a few teachers in high school who were encouraging, saying if you work hard you can be successful, but it wasn't until I got into college that a professor recognized that I had a stutter." That was a part of his journey through stuttering, but only the beginning of recognition of a link between it and the eventual diagnosis of dyslexia.

It began during his enrollment, and eventual graduation, from Ohio Wesleyan University. "When I was a junior in college, there was a professor that was a speech professor ... he wasn't a speech pathologist; he just happened to be a professor in the Speech Department, and he recognized my language pattern and started asking what the problem was. I explained as best as I could. He said Ok, I don't know much about the particulars of stuttering, but let me see if I can help you. And so, he read some stuff about it, he introduced me to the fact that Sydney Poitier was a stutterer." That opened a door for Pitts because it gave him a connection, someone with whom he could identify and a goal toward which he could aspire. From there, the professor came up with a plan. "In his reading, he saw that a teacher had Sydney Poitier speak with rocks in his mouth. So, he had the bright idea to have me talk with pencils in my mouth in order to feel what it felt like to speak clearly. Then we worked to figure out what my triggers would be."

It would be an arduous challenge, but one for which Byron Pitts was ready. "For me, if I'm tired, if I became emotional, whether happy or sad or angry ... I might stutter. He even made list of words I struggle with most. He had me read the *New York Times* backwards, which

Chapter 5. Byron Pitts

presented its own challenges. Then he ultimately decided he forced me to take a live radio show. In his mind if I could be forced to confront it, you know ... like white knuckle it every day, then I would eventually learn to manage it. And that kind of set with how I was raised, that my mother's philosophy was work hard, play hard and [be optimistic], you can do anything. So that's been the pattern of my life."

There was another turning point in college where Pitts was able to see the connection between his stuttering and dyslexia. "I had a very good friend in college; his name is John C. McGinley, an actor." McGinley would eventually have roles in TV series, including *Scrubs*, and movies, including *Platoon* and *Wall Street*. The timing of their meeting and friendship was pivotal. "The professor recommended that we both get tested because she thought we both had learning issues. And John's family had more means than my own. He got tested and was determined to be dyslexic ... which was probably the first time I ever heard the word. Then John actually left college, but I didn't. I couldn't afford to get the testing, nor could I afford in my own mind and mother's mind to leave college ... so like other challenges you just kind of muscle through it...."

He gives a lot of credit to that professor and to Ohio Wesleyan University in general. "In fact, she started a reading program at the college level in Ohio that still exists. It's designed to recognize students who may have learning needs. I mean certainly not all the kids who go through the program are dyslexic.... I mean it's not designed specifically for that, but it is a place you can go if you are falling behind." It taught him, among other things, that educators can play a major role in changing the lives of those with learning disabilities. "These are people that sit in positions on high ... and you know sometimes, I guess, when we sit on high we start to recognize people who need your help that don't respond to you in the traditional ways. But OWU has a wonderful heart for growing students."

His early college experience should give hope to anyone who struggles with education at any level. It was anything but perfect. In fact, he was on academic probation and faced several turning points, even considering quitting after a discouraging interaction with one of his professors. "My freshman year in college, I was on academic probation, not doing well, a midterm away from flunking out of school, and my English professor one day passed out papers and announced to the class: Congratulations, Mr. Pitts, your best work thus far: D+. Come see me after class."

Dutifully, he went to the professor's office. "It's my opinion you're

Dyslexia and the Journalist

not Ohio Wesleyan University material," he was told. "'You're wasting my time and the government's money.' That quotation has lived for a long time in my family. I was 17 years old and raised to respect authority. So, I thought if this man said I wasn't worthy, I should leave."

Next there came a fortuitous interaction.

> I left his office, went next door and began filling out the papers to withdraw from school, and I started to cry because I was mindful of what that decision would mean for me, mean for my family, the shame it would bring to my family. As I was crying, a stranger walked by. I didn't know her. She didn't know me. And she said: "Young man, what's wrong?" And I told her my story. She sat down, and she listened for about 20 minutes, said come see me the next day. Come to find out, that stranger was also an English professor at Ohio Wesleyan. Her name is Ulle Lewes. She's from the country of Estonia.

Byron Pitts had found a kindred soul in perseverance. "She was a child of World War II. So she recognized struggle. She'd endured discrimination during World War II. So, I think she recognized struggle in this young person. She stopped. She helped me. She became my unofficial advisor. In fact, she told me then, on academic probation, she said, son, someday you will write a book." Her prophecy came true. To date, Byron Pitts has written and published not one, but *two* books, *Step Out on Nothing: How Faith and Family Helped Me Conquer Life's Challenges*, in 2010, and *Be the One: Six True Stories of Teens Overcoming Hardship with Hope*, in 2018.

Ulle Lewes had become, on a desperate day in a young man's life, the one person who made the right difference at the right time, in the exactly right moment. "She was encouraging, just like my mother and other people in my life, and she planted seeds of kindness in me and optimism, and she encouraged me, she worked with me after hours. She stepped out on nothing for me and made all the difference in the world."

The other difference came in the form of a letter from his mother, the person who had most believed in him as a child and now, even more so, as an adult. The letter starts off, "Dear Mr. Brain-dead. Have you lost your mind?" Laughing at it now, Pitts recalls every word of the letter. "She goes on to say, in very choice language, very creative language, to make the case that you're not going to quit school, you're not going to give up, you're going to work your way past your problems."

As he moved forward in college, Pitts made adaptations that made life with dyslexia somewhat easier to navigate. "One of the things I learned in learning how to read was just rote, just repetition. So, for instance, the way I tackled my school work in college was to audio record, then at night for most of college.... I took notes as best I could and then when I got home, I transcribed them.... I typed them out, in most of my classes. That's how I study." Still, while in college and transitioning to his professional life, dyslexia continued to bring challenges. "I felt that I can't comprehend information as quickly as many of my peers. I've also said that I'd rather be shot at, caught in a hurricane than be given the document to read live on the air to go over."

Journalism, at first, didn't seem an intuitive choice for a young man with a stuttering problem and diagnosed dyslexia. "I wouldn't call it natural, but certainly that is one of the reasons why I gravitated to it after graduating from Ohio Wesleyan," he says. "They have a really strong print journalism school. There was a lack of respect, if not contempt, for broadcast journalism. I found it an easier medium for me for a couple of reasons: one because it's more of a team activity than I found print journalism to be and having lived in a world of sports and even music, for me it's always been a group activity. I like that about it."

For a kid who had his share of emotional upheaval in childhood, the new college graduate embraced what he sees as the "heart" behind television storytelling. "I found that broadcast journalism to me is as much about making an emotional connection as it is making a word or language connection. So, I find that easier." A lesson that couldn't be taught in school is a level of empathy, transferred from his personal disability to a broader understanding of others' problems and challenges. "You know, often times when I'm working on a story, I'll decide how I feel about it ... how it moves me before I can sit down and write about it."

As he has grown older and had children of his own, Pitts has also recognized that dyslexia is a difficult concept for those outside the dyslexic community to grasp. "Certainly it is something that people can read about and have heard about, and I think most people are now familiar with the word, but they don't fully understand it," he says. "If it's not your issue people don't pick it up." At the same time, it's a personal goal. "I want to believe that most people are empathetic, but you're only empathetic to things your senses respond to. If someone's blind, if someone is physically handicapped in some way that you can see and hear, something that's tangible, then people are all in. But being dyslexic, having the challenge or problem with literacy, you can't really see that. You have to experience that, spend time with sometime to see it and then be able to respond to it in some way."

Interestingly, Byron Pitts has six children, two biological and four adopted. None are dyslexic, which goes against the grain, somewhat, of

Dyslexia and the Journalist

how dyslexia is often passed on from parent to child. According to one study, "it's not uncommon for a child with dyslexia to have an immediate family member who also has this condition. Also, it's not unusual for two or more children in a family to have this type of learning disability." Other research suggests that "if either a father or a mother is dyslexic their sons have approximately a 75% risk of being dyslexic, whilst girls will have a 25% chance." That doesn't mean heredity is a guarantee a child will be dyslexic, but the predisposition is high, especially in boys.

For Byron Pitts, genetics didn't come into play, but "grit," a term often used to describe toughing it out, did—and still does. He began practicing journalism during an internship at a North Carolina TV station. After college, he set out for the career he now has in television news. There were many stops along the way, including local stations in Orlando, Tampa, Boston, and Atlanta; he also spent two years as a military reporter for a station in Portsmouth, Virginia. In those early days, despite all the hard work to combat his stuttering, at times it persisted.

There was the time during a TV live shot when he was covering a case of government corruption. To avoid stuttering, he prepared and rehearsed what he had to say. But when the moment arrived for him to go live on air, "rather than hearing the introduction I expected on the corruption story, the anchor asked me a question about the weather. I froze. I was unable to react quickly to the unexpected question. In trying to respond, I stuttered. I intended to say that it had started to snow when we first arrived this morning. But it came out as 's-s-s-s-s-snow.' I looked at my feet to try to kick-start my brain."

It's something that sticks with Byron Pitts to this day, a memory he often refers to during interviews. "That night I ate my dinner alone in an edit suite and watched that live shot over and over again. I made a copy on VHS tape and took it home so I could watch it again. I wanted to see if there was a way to prevent something like that from ever happening again. But the shame has never left me."

Despite the setback, his big break came in 1997, when he was hired as a correspondent for CBS Newspath, a video service that provides stories to local CBS news stations. He was named a national correspondent for the *CBS Evening News* in 1998, soon after moving up to the position of chief national correspondent. He was one of the network's lead reporters during the September 11 attacks, work for which he was awarded a national Emmy. It was his second Emmy, having won the first in 1999 for coverage of the Chicago train wreck. Other notable reporting achievements include: covering the Iraq War, during which he came

Chapter 5. Byron Pitts

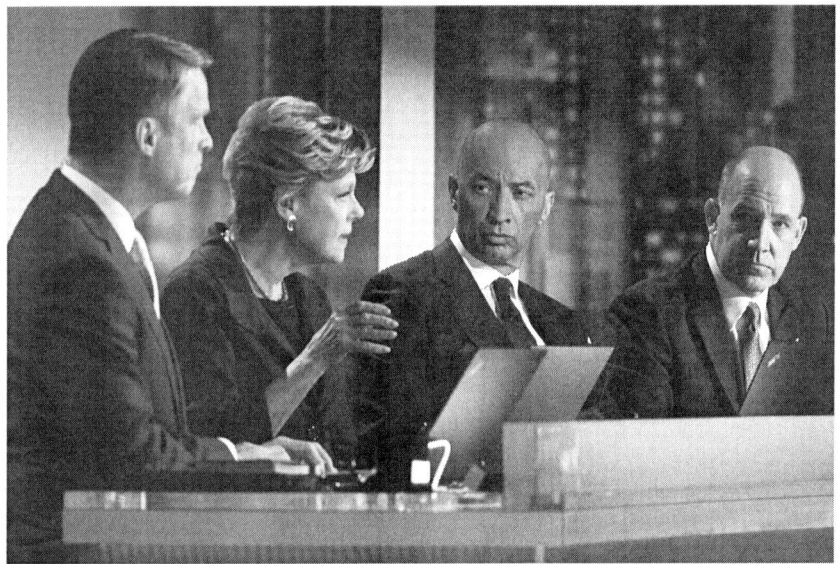

Byron Pitts during coverage of the 2018 midterm election, with the late Cokie Roberts (courtesy ABC News/Lorenzo Bevilaqua).

under fire while reporting on the fall of Saddam Hussein's statue; Hurricane Katrina; the war in Afghanistan; and the refugee crisis in Kosovo.

He is also the recipient of four Associated Press awards and six regional Emmys, all measures of high achievement in the field of journalism in general and specifically in broadcast journalism. The National Association of Black Journalists also honored him in 2002.

Not bad for a kid with dyslexia who once heard an "expert" tell his mother he was "retarded" and should be institutionalized. Not bad at all.

In the process, he has become an inspiration to those who are told "never" over and over again.

Since he was eighteen, Byron Pitts's dream was to be on the most watched television news magazine show in history: *60 Minutes*. In a 2015 speech to students at North Carolina State University, Pitts recalled the experience of visiting the show's set. "I would go and walk around the place," he said. "I was measuring for the drapes and deciding which office would be mine."

> My prayer since I was eighteen was, "Lord, make me good enough to work at *60 Minutes* someday." Those are the exact words.... My prayers were answered. My faith constantly reminds me that God can see beyond our greatest desires for ourselves.

Dyslexia and the Journalist

That dream was achieved during his fifteen-year tenure at CBS News, before moving to ABC News in 2013, where he co-anchors the network's *Nightline* broadcast, as well as contributing to its other programming, including *Good Morning America* and *World News Tonight*. Along the way, while actualizing his own potential, he has formulated opinions on how the news media can do a better job of covering the "silent disability" of dyslexia.

At the basic level, he says, the solutions aren't very complex.

> They are simple things. I think if one of the mantras of journalism is to shed light in dark places, certainly there is lots of misinformation and lack of knowledge in this space when it comes to dyslexia.... Certainly, I know when I was a child, and even as a young adult, there was a direct line between a person's intellect and their challenges with dyslexia. There's an assumption that if you were dyslexic or had any traces of it, that you were somehow less than intellectual. So, if society tells you that you're less than, then you spend a good part of your time hiding. You live in shame. It causes you to hide and wear a mask; it causes you not to seek help. So, I certainly think the media can always play a role in shedding light in places to removing the stigma in things. I think it's an easy place to start.

With that as a start, he hopes some myths and misinformation surrounding dyslexia will be dispelled.

In his own workplace, first at CBS News and now at ABC, Byron Pitts says he works hard, on an individual basis, to reshape the image of what a dyslexic is ... and isn't. Coworkers in the newsrooms where he is and has been are often surprised to learn he is dyslexic. "Certainly, at a point in my professional life, anyone who worked with me knew what some of my challenges were, I think." He laughs, remembering the reaction of several colleagues. "I think the reaction was what I expected, the unspoken reaction was 'huh ... I always thought you were bright ... you look normal.'" His former colleague, the *60 Minutes* correspondent Sharyn Alfonsi, recalls the day she learned Byron Pitts was dyslexic. "As a correspondent, you have to consume so much reading and comprehend it in a short period of time, and I was amazed that he figured out how to do that and never missed a beat! I had no idea. He was a rising star at the network; nothing seemed to hold him back."[6]

He also recognizes where that comes from in others. The experiences of Sir Richard Branson, among other high-profile dyslexics, resonate. Branson, he is reminded, would often hear similar statements from those outside the dyslexic community. Branson once recalled that dyslexia was like a rash—something that others, when they learned of his

Chapter 5. Byron Pitts

dyslexia, would react along the lines of "well, you've clearly healed yourself and gotten rid of it." Branson is someone who has written about how his dyslexia "got me to where I am today." Similar to Pitts's experience with the education "expert" at age twelve, Branson, at fifteen, was told by his school headmaster that he would one day end up in prison (although, to be fair, the other option, the headmaster relayed, was as a billionaire).

The road to the top of his field has been a long one, and, in the process, some things from his earlier life have been left behind, sports being one of them. The interesting connection Pitts observed between the "language" of calling plays as a quarterback, the rhythm of music, and the cadence of the spoken word has never left him, and there's still a connection he'd one day like to revisit. He has never coached a sport, but it's an aspiration. "I would love to! My life ambition is to be a little league football coach when I retire. But you know like a lot of people I have been so preoccupied with building my career and raising my family there's not much room for anything else."

He has done a different kind of coaching, however, in the community, both where he grew up and beyond. "I do a lot of public speaking about literacy. Certainly because of the nature of my job I get to go to speak to different organizations from corporations to school settings to faith organizations. I give about twenty speeches a year." It is both personal and a broader mission, he says. "I support students at my all boys' Catholic school. I support students there through scholarships with monies I give, either students who come from low-income families or students who perform poorly academically. I weave into my speeches my unlikely story of success."

In addition, he has contributed to the success of others who face the same or similar challenges. One is a little girl he met during a visit to a Baltimore public school. Her name is Pilar. She asked him one question that he says left a lasting impression: "Where do you hide when the world hurts too much?" Pilar, like Pitts, was diagnosed with learning disorders, but, unlike him, was abandoned by her mother when she was ten. Over the years, he stayed in touch with her, becoming a mentor. He is proud to say that, through her own hard work and the support of the right people, Pilar graduated high school and went on to college.[7]

He also had the opportunity to have his "warrior mother," Clarice, see all he had accomplished, before her death in 2011. As he told an audience at North Carolina State University in 2018, for most of her seventy-seven years, his mom had been the one in charge of the family. At the end of her life, Pitts and his siblings joined together to care for her. "It was an awful time for my mother and my family," he recalls. "But we got through it." He remembered her vibrant personality, her love of politics, most of all her sense of humor. She was the one everyone in the family went to for advice. Given her son's dyslexia, one thing Byron Pitts will always revere about his mother was her own love of reading.

Clarice Pitts, he says, lost so much of herself, that personality, that love of reading and learning, when dementia set in four years before her passing. There were days she wouldn't speak a single word, and others when she would tear into her children suddenly and impulsively. Still, the Pitts family never got overwhelmed, because, he says, everyone had a role to play and did so lovingly. His sister lived close by in North Carolina, and, between them, brothers and sisters, cousins and uncles set up a detailed caregiving schedule. "My mother had a small army taking care of her," he says. "She was never left by herself—not once."

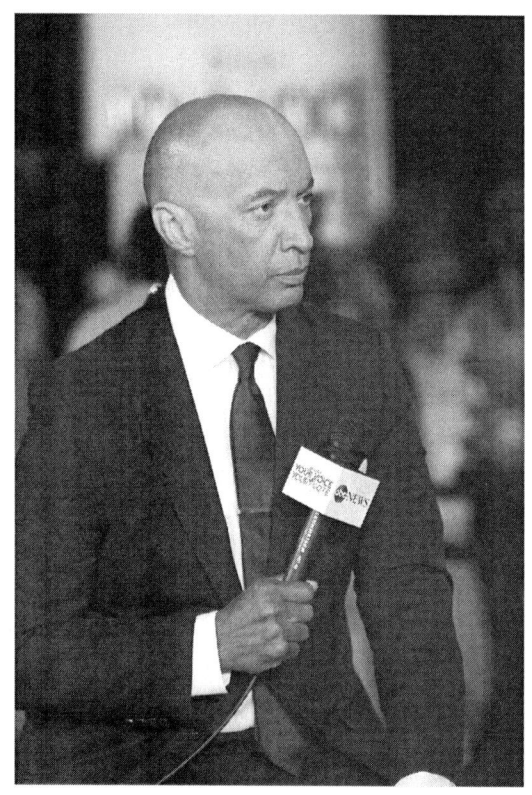

Byron Pitts during coverage of a 2020 Democratic debate, 2020 (courtesy ABC News).

His mother had taught him well and life had come full circle since she had cared so deeply for him. Still, after her passing, with all he had done to facilitate her care, Byron Pitts felt it still was not enough. He wished he had been more patient. He wished, he once said, that "I had taken the time to say 'mom, you want some ice cream? Ok, let's do that.'" Instead, he adds, "I was clinging on to who she was instead of embracing who she was in this moment."

There was so much he had learned from her that translated into

Chapter 5. Byron Pitts

his adult life. There's an expression he says he picked up while embedded with Marines during the Gulf War. It's called "Embrace the suck." It means to "accept that something is unpleasant and unavoidable ... and then deal with it." That's what he and his family did. "Alzheimer's and dementia sucked—there's nothing good about it. But it is what is," he adds. "It doesn't go away, but it changes your attitude about how you deal with it," like dyslexia.

As he learned more about dyslexia, he became the advocate for others that his mother had been for him. He did his own research and learned some startling statistics. "According to the National Center for Family Literacy," he discovered, "more than 30 million adults in the United States cannot read or comprehend information at the most basic level." He pauses to let that number sink in. "When I think about that number, it reminds me how offended I am when some suggest we in the news should 'dumb it down.' How about we elevate our work so people can understand it, and be inspired by it?"

Inspiration is what defines Byron Pitts, both being inspired and inspiring others. "I hope my story teaches or reinforces the value of optimism and hard work. I heard the actor Laurence Fishburne say not long ago, 'It's not what you do, it's how you do it that matters.' I like that. I've always worked to do the best I can. I've spent many hours obsessing about many things, but I don't spend much energy trying to be like someone else. I figure God made me the way he wanted me. My job is to just be the very best Byron Pitts I can be."[8]

He once told students at Georgetown University that at one point in his early schooling he was banished from the classroom. "I remember when I became [one of] what was called the basement boys, where you would send kids who [had] either academic or behavior problems." Yes, he and the other "slow kids" were sent, literally, to the basement, almost like being put in a cell and forgotten.

As for becoming a journalist with dyslexia and a stuttering problem, he doesn't see the connection as at all unusual. "One reason I became a journalist was because as a child who couldn't read, I knew what it was to be voiceless; no one asked my opinion. My opinion didn't matter," Pitts says. "Strength only comes from struggle in life, and there [are] always things you can learn," Pitts said of overcoming his severe stuttering and coping with his dyslexia. "It taught me to think before I speak, which as a journalist is a good skill to have."[9]

At every opportunity, he shares, especially with those who are dyslexic, a mantra of hope and perseverance: "Embrace the gift that has

Dyslexia and the Journalist

made you mentally tough. Know that you have gotten to this point in your life, in part because you ARE mentally tough! Your work ethic is five times more than anyone else. Actually, it's persistence." And, he adds that your story can be an inspiration to others. "Ask if you are explaining to others all the time, to anyone you meet, that dyslexia is a neurological disorder of the brain and that, while we learn differently, we're just as capable."

Chapter 6

Robyn Curnow

"You never forget that early humiliation of being the last to finish in class or having a teacher throw a book at you."—Robyn Curnow

Robyn Curnow is an anchor for CNN and CNN–International, where she first began reporting from London in 2001. Previously, she reported for both the BBC and the South African Broadcasting Corporation.

Like many parents, CNN's Robyn Curnow didn't realize she had dyslexia until her child was diagnosed with it. It not only helped Curnow make sense of her own struggles growing up; it also helped her realize "that many things I was good at were also because of dyslexia." It's a difficult story for any parent to share, and being in the public eye as a journalist can make it feel particularly harrowing. Throughout her life, however, Curnow has established an important mantra for those who know little or nothing about the condition: there's an upside to dyslexia.

Robyn Curnow was born in Australia and raised in Johannesburg, South Africa. She is the eldest child, with two brothers. When you hear her speak, it is evident that Robyn has a lot of pride in and love for her country, beginning with the energy in South Africa's largest city that makes it an exciting place to be. Johannesburg is where she went to school and started her broadcasting career. It's a path that would one day lead to a job at the South African Broadcasting Corporation during one of the most pivotal times in her home nation's history, at England's BBC, and, currently, since 2001, at CNN. In addition, she earned a prestigious master's degree from Cambridge University in the United Kingdom.[1]

Along the way, she has written for *Vogue* magazine, *Marie-Claire*, the *International Herald Tribune*, and the *Washington Post*. She has interviewed world leaders, including former U.S. presidents Bill Clinton, George W. Bush, and Barack Obama, as well as the anti–Apartheid freedom fighter and former South African president Nelson Mandela.

Dyslexia and the Journalist

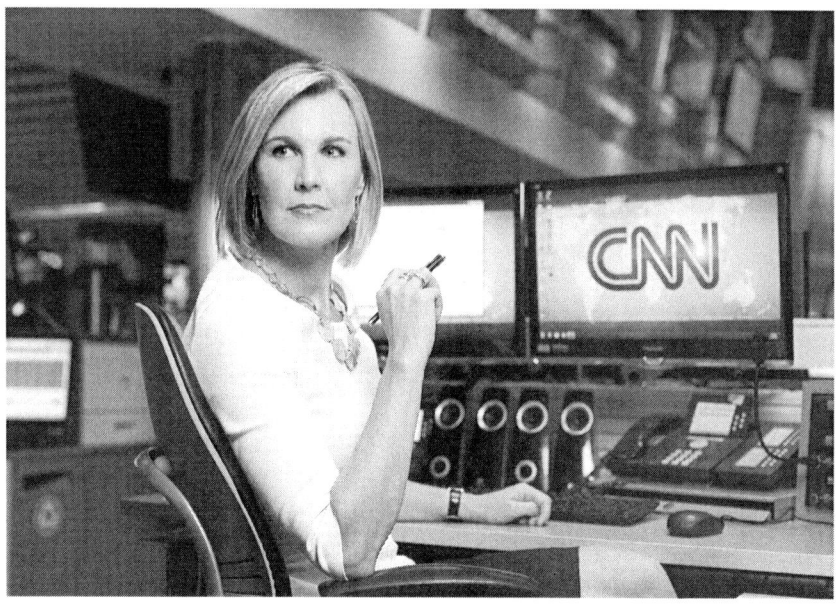

Robyn Curnow at work at CNN in Atlanta (courtesy CNN).

She has reported from Cuba on the occasion of Fidel Castro's death and on human rights violations in nations around the globe—pretty impressive for a woman who was told by her teachers that she would amount to nothing.[2]

Most recently, she has made her home in Atlanta, Georgia, home to CNN's international headquarters. "In 2014 we moved to Atlanta," she relays. "I have two daughters.... My youngest daughter, while in kindergarten and through first grade, showed several red flags." Instead of writing "dog," she'd write "bog." She wrote "b" and "d" in inverse directions and got tripped up between "m," "n," and "w." That wasn't all. "I watched as she learned a word like 'C-A-T' and then forget it the next day. Words, letters, and sounds became elusive to her, like grasping at bubbles blowing in the wind."[3]

Words and sounds are the stock and trade of journalists, so it is not surprising that her youngest daughter's symptoms resonated with her. In fact, the path to recognizing her own dyslexia went through her daughter. "It was only a few years ago that I realized I was dyslexic," she says. "It kind of coincided with my younger child's path to literacy, as she was diagnosed with dyslexia at age of 6 or 7 ... and in trying to educate myself about her.... I suddenly realized, oh that explains a lot—I'm dyslexic too! It was a relief to know I was dyslexic as an adult, it was also quite a stunning piece of self-knowledge because it explained so much...."[4]

"Remembering back, my daughter struggled with nursery rhymes, as well as remembering them," she says, and her daughter also struggled with tying her shoes. "In addition, she started getting reluctant to read back words to me in the early learning phase. For example, one year we put out at Christmas several books, as it's always a special time, and she started getting nervous about seeing them."

The decision was made to turn toward testing to help determine the problem and, potentially, find treatment. "When we got her tested and they went over all the tests, they told us it was dyslexia. I really had no idea and didn't know what it was.... I mean, I was very ignorant in terms of exactly what dyslexia was. I thought it was just reading backwards. I really didn't understand the nuances of what it was, and the teacher said to me—you know that it's genetic. And then I went... 'Oh of course, my father was dyslexic!'"

It wasn't instant recognition.

> I immediately didn't make the connection with myself, I made it with my dad, because my dad was an amazing man, but I think he was almost illiterate when he died. He really struggled to read at all. Our stories at home often referred to the traumas of his schooling. He would talk about being beaten at school for not remembering poems. They would lock him away and punish him, and he failed, he didn't make it through high school. I think my dad's stuttering came from the fact that as a child in early learning he couldn't read, he couldn't write and then the priests in the Catholic school would hit him on the knuckles with a ruler or they would beat him. So, I think my dad's stutter was an outcome of the dyslexia.

Robyn understands now that there are often connections between stuttering and dyslexia, and she links many of her father's experiences to dyslexia. "Another fact, my dad was creative and artistic and I think those are very dyslexic things. I often say that his granddaughters managed to have this extraordinary experience in America by going to the Schneck School (one of the top schools for dyslexic students in America), for example, and by being remediated and supported the way my youngest daughter is now." The thought often crosses her mind of how different her father's life might have been. "You know it would have been something where he would have had a very different life if he had had that education." And there's this poignant reminder of a moment long ago involving her dad and her daughter. "I have a memory of him trying to read a story to my eldest daughter, but really he wasn't reading it, he was only telling a story about the pictures."

Though he wasn't proficient at reading, Robyn says, "My dad was very good at telling us stories. I would very often talk with my dad and he was very, very keen that I got a good education. He was the one that pushed for us to go to private school. We didn't have a lot of money, but my dad was insistent, and particularly with me. He kept a very close eye on me in terms of making sure that I went to private school, and it was once I found the right school that I managed to thrive." It wasn't easy. "The first school that I went to, I had a lot of traumatic experiences; it was, again, in a Catholic school. And interestingly, I think he might have recognized that the nuns weren't particularly gracious for kids who didn't fit into the mold."

The lessons learned from her dad stuck. "It was interesting the way I fought for my daughter in terms of education and remediation, and that's because I understand how much dyslexia held my father back as an opportunity. So, in many ways I've used dyslexia to create resilience in ways that, instead, gave him weakness." Now, knowing her dad was dyslexic helped chart the course for her youngest child.

"We sent our youngest to the Schenck School ... widely regarded as one of the top schools for dyslexic students in the United States. How fortunate that it was located here in Atlanta. The school's strategy is focused on accelerated remediation of dyslexia using the highly effective Orton-Gillingham approach." That means that while reading and writing are central to the school's curriculum, the school also has a comprehensive educational program that "helps all students develop intellectually and prepare them to reenter mainstream schools successfully."

Parents of dyslexic children, whether themselves dyslexic or not, are also educated on the condition. "There were a number of educational parent talks at my daughter's school, to help parents learn more about dyslexia so they would have a better understanding of what it would be like if they were to have dyslexia." One, in particular, left a lasting memory.

> I went to this one parent lecture that was held in the school cafeteria, and all of us were sitting at long tables with benches. The school teachers wanted to give parents a sense of what dyslexia was like, to have a bad teacher, or a teacher who didn't understand dyslexia. The teacher walked in and out around the tables and chairs quickly and she was very loud and she was talking very fast and giving a lot of instructions very quickly. "Turn to page 26 quickly ... you gotta go to this Section B." It was fast, quick instructions

with way too much detail that you get a dyslexic kid. So already you're feeling bamboozled with information being jabbed at you! And then she said in front of you, "Okay, and now in front of you, you have a pamphlet worksheet. I need you to do it in ten minutes. You have to be finished. There's a time limit."[5]

The experience reminded Robyn of her own childhood schooling, the stress especially.

> So, already you have the pressure of this time limit and all this information that's being given to you and you're trying to process this. And then I opened up the worksheet and there were a lot of visual spatial activities and she then said, "write with your left hand, or your opposite dominant hand." They did this because they wanted to give you a sense of the disconnect between your hand and your brain. So, I'm writing left-handed and you kind of had to connect various things, and all the while … the teacher was continuing to talk incessantly and talking over you and then starts praising those who are doing it right. It was such an interesting simulation of bombarding people, where the information keeps on coming … you can't concentrate. You're timed with limits, and then she starts praising other people and you start feeling unconfident already because you're not doing it fast enough. I was moving and I was trying to connect the dots, linking up things and I was really trying to concentrate. Then, the teacher yells "Okay, time's up!" I sort of pulled back and looked at my paper and just thought, "God that must look awful. I remember what that was like!"

The feelings came rushing back, all at once, and the feeling was intense.

> I was really feeling overwhelmed, because it takes you back. The yelling teachers, the pressure had created a situation that was an overstimulation, clearly representative of duress. Then one of the mothers who was sitting next to me … looked over at my work and laughed out loud exclaiming something to the effect of "Ohhh my God, what did you do!" It was so visceral, that sense of failure, that sense of pressure and the sense of judgment! I felt this so deep down in myself, it was like some sort of weird regression where I felt like I was six again. I started crying. It was embarrassing, I tried to hide behind my glasses but it was such a raw emotion that I think it was such a very good teaching tool for many parents who perhaps weren't dyslexic but they wouldn't have understood the pressure. But, I do think for a lot of the parents who were dyslexic it was a **terrible reminder** [emphasis added] of what it was like at school where you didn't have the luxury of being somewhere like the Schneck School.

That day helped Robyn Curnow work through her own preconceptions about dyslexia, leading to an important realization.

> In those days I was still sort of fascinated and would say "Oh, do you think I'm dyslexic?" I mean, I know how difficult this was to process, and that was

a diagnosis if ever there was one. It was such a powerful moment, such a self-reflection and self-agony. I went back to that teacher who had done it and sat with her. I said, "You wouldn't believe how awful that felt to me, and it was like I regressed." She said, "I know, and I'm so sorry that happened to you and you had that reaction, but so many teachers are still like that today. Across the world, your experience has not improved for many children." I said, I know. The two of us then worked through what dyslexia is, my strengths and weaknesses. And so, it was a very cathartic process. This was a great simulation, and a very good reminder to me. In fact, this is one of the reasons why I have been speaking about it.

Thinking back, it wasn't only her father's experience that brought about Robyn's epiphany regarding dyslexia.

My mother was extremely, extremely determined that the school had made the wrong assessment on me. She knew I was bright and that I could recite stories back to her, but she wasn't buying the teacher when she said this child is going to be a good wife or mother one day, don't expect much for her. Thank God I had a mother who fought for me! I was very lucky to have my mother fight for me when I was five, six years old. The biggest thing she did was to boost my confidence. I think that ... the most successful dyslexics are the ones that have had somebody who not necessarily taught them to read, but gave a sense of self, despite the fact that you're often going to school and failing and making mistakes, constantly picking yourself up and having to go back again.

Her mother's faith in her was also a game changer for a young girl struggling in what must have seemed like a rigged game. "If you know within yourself there's somebody that thinks that you're fantastic, it makes the biggest difference ... you just need one person to be your North Star. That can take you very far to have that North Star." Eventually, she says, "you get to a point where you have to do for yourself, as you can't bring your mother into the classroom anymore. I think the role of the parent in terms of being a fighter is very important in that very early stage."

Sometimes that means making the tough choices for your child.

They kept me back a year, I repeated a year and that was what helped me where I got the extra time in a school that was focused on sports and less academics. I didn't feel like I was getting that pressure. By the time you are ten or eleven or a teenager, you have to fight your own battles. You can't go to into school and come back to mom and say "I didn't' make it in my science test" because the teachers aren't going to take that on. So, if you have that very early learning confidence boost and then the confidence comes also from your home, and then there's that resilience that I'm big on.... I don't

Chapter 6. Robyn Curnow

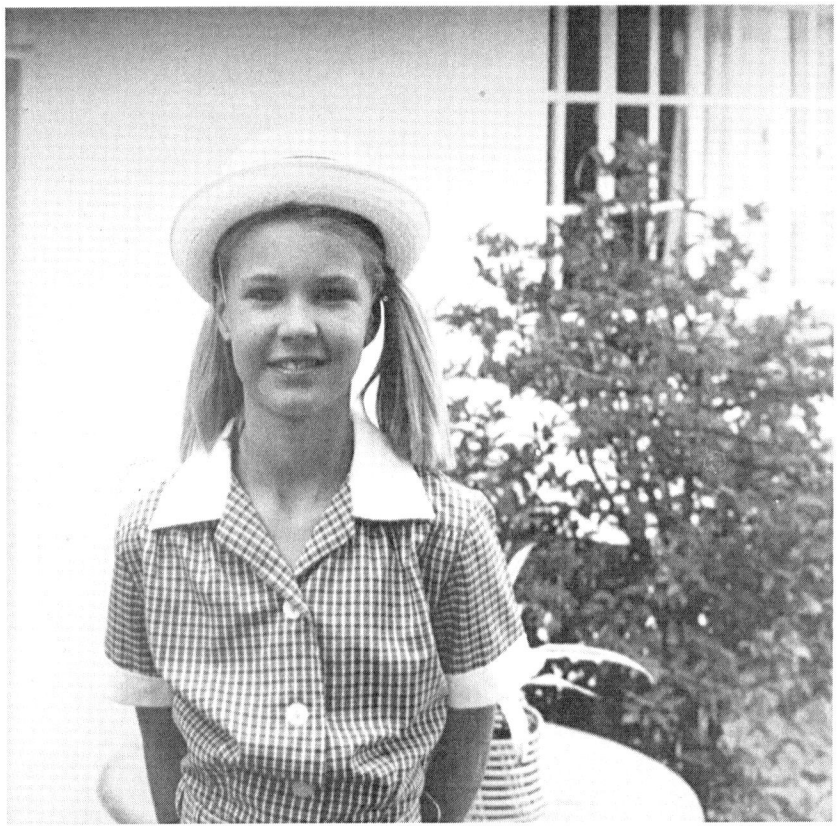

Robyn Curnow in 1980, on the first day of school in South Africa (courtesy Robyn Curnow).

think I would be here today if I didn't have dyslexia because I had to learn very early on that I was on my own.

Her major motivation was to have opportunities outside the nation where she grew up, South Africa, which at the time was torn by the racial divide of Apartheid. "The only person that was going to pull me through and get me out of suburban Apartheid South Africa was me. So, it was my own sense of ambition that I think I was fired up. I knew that I didn't want to be the last kid in the class. That burn comes from understanding what it's like to fail and make mistakes every day and knowing you still have to walk in and fix it. So, again, knowing that you have to work doubly hard, but you are on your own—no one picks you up."

There were things at which Robyn excelled or, at the very least, performed better than in strict academic subjects. "For me growing up in school, I was involved in [other nonacademic subjects] such as, I did art in school and studied art and I matriculated toward art and the history of art. I painted and then I also studied the history of art at the university. I continued to paint, and I paint to relax with acrylics and I still do that with my girls."

Connecting to her daughters came not only through the portal of dyslexia, but also, in the case of her eldest daughter, stuttering. "The stutter was triggered … in 2015, soon after we moved to the United States from South Africa. I do not know why she suddenly struggled to speak, but it was probably the combination of the stresses of the move, fellow students teasing about her South African accent, and genetics. My daughter's stutter gut punched me because my dad also stuttered." It's a powerful memory. "One of my earliest memories is of hearing him answer the phone and struggle to say his name. From then on, I would rush to the phone whenever it rang, trying to get there first so I could answer and save dad from the ordeal of having to say 'Hello.' We children were told not to interrupt my father when he stuttered, so I remember just standing there, looking up at him, patiently waiting for him to stammer out the words."

Her father died nearly ten years ago. Luckily, his granddaughter, as relayed above, received the help that he never had. "Not showing our heartache, or frustration, when [she] is laboring through a sentence or story is difficult. But telling a child while she is mid-stutter to 'slow down' or 'take a breath' is the worst thing someone can do. After a few false starts with speech therapists that had no idea how to deal with a newly stuttering seven-year-old girl, we discovered a speech pathologist in Atlanta, where we live. The pathologist, himself a stutterer, guided my daughter through the rough spots and trained her to recognize when she got stuck."

As we've seen in the other journalists in this book, stuttering is a common trait in many dyslexics. "Stuttering can be a speech block in your throat, on your tongue, or on your lips. Stuttering is also cyclical. Sometimes, my husband and I would notice [our daughter] speaking more fluidly and rejoice. Within days she would be battling her words again," says Curnow. Gradually her daughter learned exercises and tricks for "phrasing" her sentences. "Phrasing has become a euphemism in our house for speaking clearly and smoothly. Also, she has learned to help herself. Unlike my dad, whom I remember endlessly pushing through his stutters, trying hard to finish a word, [our daughter] has learned how to stop herself and recognize where she's stuck. Throat? Lips? Or tongue? She'll then try to repeat the word or sentence cleanly. When that happens, we say, 'Hey, good pickup.'"[6]

"That's easier said than done, as countless stutterers have found. People can stutter in any language and in any culture. More men stutter than women. Often, the earlier a stutter starts, the more likely the child is to grow out of it," Robyn learned. "For older stutterers, it's about managing their own Devil's Snare. Our [daughter] spoke flawlessly in front of her school assembly last spring, beautifully reading the school's character pledge in front of hundreds of fellow students, teachers and, as if the pressure weren't enough, former president Jimmy Carter, a special guest of the school. My husband and I cried from our seats on the bleachers at the back of the school gym."

These are moments in which to revel.

> I have watched in wonder as [our daughter] and, to some extent, my dad (who became less handicapped by his stutter as he aged) dealt with their sentences going rogue. Their resilience is repeated in private and public by so many other stammerers. Former vice president Joe Biden apparently had a stutter. So does the singer Ed Sheeran. When former General Electric CEO Jack Welch was a child, he once wrote, his mother told him that he stuttered because he was so smart—that his tongue could not keep up with his brain. We told [our daughter] something similar before we found her help. Words are powerful. Getting them out, for some, is empowering.

Whether it's stuttering or dyslexia, now, as a mother, Robyn Curnow believes strongly in the power of diagnosis and treatment, and the sooner the better.

> My early school days were also a struggle, but unlike my daughter, my issue wasn't identified and remediated because my teachers just did not understand I had a common learning disorder. They just thought I was not very clever. I was so bad at writing that my second grade teacher created an extra level of failure in one particularly brutal report card. She felt that "Very Poor" just didn't seem to capture my lack of aptitude. So, in neat handwriting inserted into the report, she created an additional "Extremely Weak" category, just for me. The same teacher got so frustrated with my lack of progress with math word problems she threw the textbook at me during class.

Can you imagine? This was Robyn Curnow's reality. There was nothing fantastical about it. It *was* real. "As I look back at my childhood and surviving through school, I realized that I learned very early on that I had to be *resilient*." The word comes up consistently in Robyn's conversation and her writing about dyslexia. "You learn to be resilient … and

Dyslexia and the Journalist

also to be an extremely hard worker because you literally have to work double time to keep up with everybody else. But one has to also be kind of sneaky, you find alternative paths, you kind of plan ahead to make up for your weaknesses. In many ways by the time you finish school, you're quite prepared for the real world, you become a bit of a street fighter!"

It's a process of navigation, and few people know better than Robyn Curnow how to manage the school environment. "To make it through school, many dyslexics wrangle and hustle. At some stage you learn, haphazardly, or with the help of a patient and dedicated teacher or parent, to 'decode' language. I only realized I was dyslexic as an adult, when my young daughter was diagnosed with the condition. Dyslexia is genetic, and her diagnosis explained all my early academic struggles. My mother doggedly helped me to learn and, perhaps just as importantly, she constantly boosted my self-esteem."

Her own experience has taught her a great deal beyond reading. "We also cobble together coping strategies, classroom tricks and alternative ways of thinking to get to the same destination as everyone else. Many dyslexics learn to play to our individual strengths." Clearly, her undiagnosed dyslexia did not hold her back. "When I got accepted into Cambridge University for a Master of Philosophy degree in International Relations, I remember wishing I could find that book-throwing teacher. I had shown her, and myself, that I was not 'Extremely Weak.'"

As an aside, that same teacher who had thrown a book at her once told Robyn's mother that she was only fit to be a wife and mother. It's something she remembers and repeats to this day and has often imagined going back to meet that teacher again—and confront her with the success she's mastered. At the same time, she prefers to focus on her strengths, something it took years for her to recognize and accept.

> I think for me, my strengths with school ... and at times it felt like there weren't many ... were that I had an imagination and I was very good at general knowledge, picking up useless pieces of information. I was very interested in the outside world and if you think about the fact that I was living in Apartheid South Africa in the 1980s, the country was burning, there was no outlet to independent news. There was one state station that gave propaganda. The white community was both insular and ignorant and I felt trapped by being in a circumstance of living a life in a society that I knew was wrong.

Because opportunities for unbiased information were limited, it drove her toward wanting to know more. "We didn't have access to international news, we didn't have access to international magazines, or

Chapter 6. Robyn Curnow

we didn't see things like *Vogue* magazine or any music videos. Living in South Africa during the 1980s was a bit like living in Moscow in the '80s because of the isolation. We were very, very closed off, and it wasn't just closed off from the outside world ... white suburban middle-class people were cut off from black communities in Africa."

The feeling of isolation was a spark, she says.

> I felt incredibly claustrophobic and I think in many ways my dyslexia helped make me be creative, curious and also trying to see beyond what is immediately in front of you. I think that's what defines me. I could have tried, but my spelling was bad and I wasn't the best writer in the class; still, I knew there was a world out there that I needed to explore and I always, starting as a young teenager, I wanted to get out. So I used books, and I would try and read as much as I could. I would read slowly, but I knew that I needed to get out there. So journalism for me was an exit strategy. I always wanted to write, and I always wanted to write as a way of getting away. I always saw writing as a way of escaping. I realized that writing and journalism could take me away from the ordinariness of suburban Apartheid South Africa. It was my magic carpet.

Quite by accident and timing, that magic carpet was journalism, though she had reservations at first. "I wanted the spelling not to take away from the writing of long articles, but the remedy was TV journalism. They started to open up TV news and I landed right at a sweet spot in South Africa." Television news came naturally. "It was being able to tell stories visually in Mandela's South Africa and I got out around South Africa, and I got out to see perspectives. So, here I was being a reporter for the South African Broadcasting Corporation (SABC) from 1995, just as democracy hit. I explored and I was seeing South Africa and showing it to South Africans on the national news, but with the healthy dyslexic perspective, which was [that] we all need to see differently. Because we all needed to see that the South Africa before then was wrong."

She developed a specialty in the right place at the right time.

> I basically just told stories for many years about South Africa and did this through the Nelson Mandela and Thabo Mbeki presidency. I went to the townships and shared stories with the people. It was a very powerful time in South Africa's history that I was part of. Like I shared, there was one news outlet and it was the state newscast. There was no other news; it was the eight o'clock at night English news bulletin. This was an extraordinary time under the new South Africa led by Mandela. In many ways, I got to tell the story of South Africa's rebirth to South Africans on the news within little two-minute segments that were honed down to the most important aspects, such as connecting with people and making it universal, understanding the

Dyslexia and the Journalist

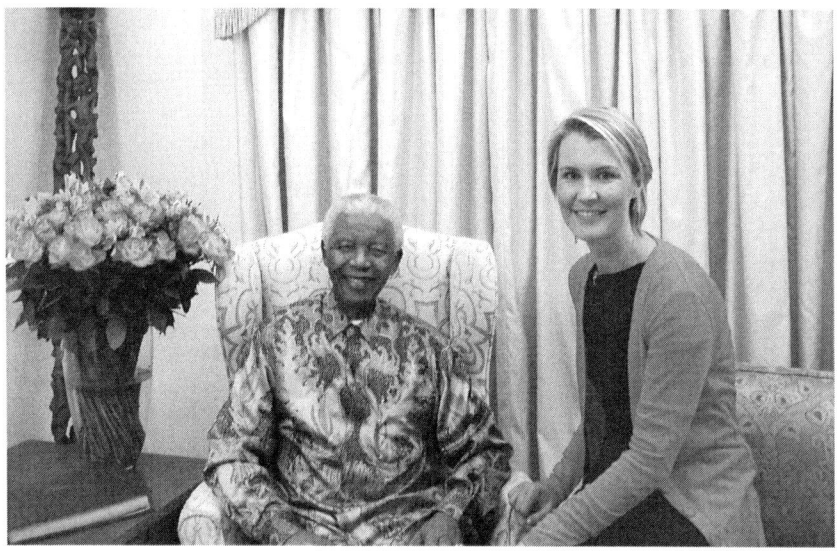

Robyn Curnow interviewing Nelson Mandela in 2008, on his ninetieth birthday (courtesy Robyn Curnow).

thread of the story, so that white middle-class girl was connecting the story of the rural areas. I was telling all of the stories. It was the perfect, perfect, perfect cocktail, showing my dyslexic strengths in many ways.

All this was accomplished against the backdrop of a young reporter who, at the time had no inkling of her disability.

Again, I didn't know I was dyslexic, but I knew I was terrible at math, I have trouble remembering things and I have trouble on immediate recall on stuff, but I'm very good if I see something, as the visual images trigger me. I knew what I was not good at, and so after school I managed to concentrate on where I was good at those things, which was also the first degree I took. It was in international relations, and political science and English, but it really was storytelling. So, as soon as I left for school, I didn't have to do math, foreign languages, and I didn't have to fit in with the structures of school. You know, going to university completely liberated me because I could do international relations and political science as it is about storytelling and the way the world works, and English literature is about stories as well. I very quickly realized that I could move towards something of a career built on my strengths.

"Harnessing creativity" is a phrase Robyn uses to describe what dyslexics share in common. "It turns out 'thinking outside of the box' comes more naturally to the dyslexic brain than the propensity to spell accurately," she says, reflecting her own experience, as well as that of her daughter. "It was a relief when I realized as an adult that I am dyslexic. What was even more liberating was realizing that many things I was good at were also because of dyslexia." She points to famous dyslexics as examples. "Each dyslexic has a different set of skills, and weaknesses, but there's a pattern of commonality that links people like Galileo, Pablo Picasso and Julia Child. Dyslexics often think in pictures and can see multi-dimensionally, which is why becoming an architect, gardener, chef and astronomer are careers that dyslexics gravitate toward."

She also sees the juxtaposition of dyslexia and writing as somewhat counterintuitive to some, but entirely understandable once people understand that dyslexia can generate creativity. "Paradoxically, dyslexics struggle to write, but are often excellent authors, such as Roald Dahl and Agatha Christie. They have 'vivid imaginations and are highly creative,' according to Made By Dyslexia, which acknowledges 9 in 10 dyslexics have poor spelling, punctuation and grammar, but many are great writers."[7]

She sees that trend in her own chosen career of TV news, a field requiring a good amount of writing.

> You know the funny thing is I didn't choose television. I didn't even choose journalism to come into; it kind of chose me to write for television. Particularly television news is like a dyslexic dream, because you have to write often in bold capital letters, the sentences are simple—you're writing to pictures and you need to take away all useless information. Luckily, I fell into a career that, I think, is a dyslexic dream job. In TV news, it's our job to think in pictures, because television is a visual medium.
>
> Anything that you put into a television news report has to be the real essence of the story and then, of course, there's storytelling. Generally, TV news is an amazing place to be able to trust your dyslexic instincts, which are [to] look at the big picture, identify the story, tell the story and create a narrative that is simplified so that an audience can understand the main issues. It's an amazing thing when you look back over your career and I think to myself hmmm maybe because I'm dyslexic might be the reason I can do what I'm doing in front of the camera.[8]

Like Richard Engel of NBC News, who is the subject of chapter 9, Robyn Curnow doesn't see the disadvantages to being dyslexic and working in TV news. "As a TV reporter you write brief, short scripts to pictures. This is a very helpful outlet, because you are using pictures and creating little two-and-a-half-minute movies and so you are using the combination of words and pictures—which I think is very creative."

Dyslexia and the Journalist

There's a built-in advantage. "The audience only hears and sees the report, so spelling and grammar are not as important as they are for, say, a newspaper article. Also, television news is about simplifying a lot of facts, analyzing events quickly and interpreting complex information—live on air. If you read the *Value of Dyslexia* report, you will see how those skills are hardwired into the dyslexic brain."

She isn't alone among CNN journalists with dyslexia. "My colleague Anderson Cooper told me that as a child he was sent to a 'reading doctor' after school in New York and during the summer in Long Island to help him with what he calls mild dyslexia. 'I still do have trouble confusing some letters and numbers,' he told me. I agree with him when he says it's easier to 'have stuff printed out to read instead of reading off a computer,' as I also rely heavily on the paper copies of scripts and news wires."[9]

Robyn has put her story into print in various venues where she discusses other working similarities shared with Cooper. "Like Anderson, sometimes my words and numbers get mixed up, so I make accommodations and create verbal safety nets for when I'm reading the autocue prompter. I edit long, convoluted sentences and remove complicated foreign names that are redundant and could trip me up. I avoid too many numbers. If I start to find words jumping and darting away like fireflies at night, I slow down and concentrate even harder. Or just move on to the next story. I love it when there's breaking news and we throw out the pre-written scripts and I'm required to ad lib."

Words, once the enemy, are now her valued friend.

> As a journalist, I love words. I care about what I write, think before I speak, read with delight and savor language. Part of that relationship with words comes from the fact that I respect them. My profession, more than most, teaches the value and importance of words, and their power. But sometimes I fear words too. Each word I write, or say, is hard fought and comes from deep within. I am dyslexic, which is a highly common learning disorder; an estimated 10 percent of school children around the world share this with me.... For us, language is a puzzle. Sometimes our brains cannot quite work out how those puzzle pieces fit together. But while having dyslexia can certainly be a challenge, it is neither a disability nor a measure of intelligence.[10]

Like Anderson Cooper, Robyn Curnow doesn't hide her dyslexia from others and, in fact, looks for opportunities to share her own experiences—and those of others—as inspiration. She cites actors like Orlando Bloom, who "says his dyslexia is like a superpower—that's a powerful message for any child struggling at school." And she adds

Chapter 6. Robyn Curnow

these words of caution: "Not every child struggling to read will be as well-known as some famous dyslexics—John Lennon, Albert Einstein, Henry Ford or Kiera Knightley. However, they do not need to be left behind, or relegated to the dunce corner. More teachers need to recognize the familiar signs and be able to help, all the tools to do so are out there, if you just look."

For a woman who loved her dad dearly and fretted over his stuttering, as well as having a mother who recognized the connection to her dyslexia, it's gratifying to see how much has improved for today's dyslexic students. "Viewing dyslexia as a unique set of abilities with varying patterns of strengths and challenges—instead of a one-size-fits-all learning disability—is gaining traction," she says. "Increasingly, allowances are being made for dyslexic children in the classroom. In the state of Georgia, where I live, a new law makes it mandatory for all children to be screened for dyslexia. Getting expert help early while children are still learning to read, and not reading to learn, is crucial."

While things have improved, Robyn adds that

> teachers or parents who think a child can "grow out" of dyslexia are wrong. If your child is constantly being told to try harder, write neater, or stop being lazy, then maybe you need to take them to be tested for the world's most common learning disorder. Help is everywhere. Many schools and universities give extra time on tests. Teachers don't penalize students for bad spelling when they're known to be dyslexic. Some schools even give dyslexic students a pass when it comes to having to learn a second language. Many allow pupils to listen to audiobooks instead of trying to plow through set reading books.

She gives credit to those corporations that have begun to embrace tools for dyslexics to learn. "Even big companies such as Microsoft are helping too. Microsoft just released free online dyslexia awareness training for parents and teachers, in coordination with Made By Dyslexia. Using teaching experts from two of the oldest specialized dyslexic schools in the United States and United Kingdom—the Schenck School in Atlanta and Millfield School in Somerset, England—these online videos aim to democratize dyslexic teaching. It's a free hour of expert instruction, speeches and books. Microsoft's learning tools also have incredible options for dyslexics, such as tools which read out text, break up syllables and increase spaces between lines and letters."

Robyn is also very passionate about the charity Made By Dyslexia, which is supported by the proud dyslexic Sir Richard Branson. The billionaire has gathered together a smorgasbord of powerful and creative

Dyslexia and the Journalist

people who share this learning disorder. Alongside Branson, who famously dropped out of school early, but is now a global disrupter and billionaire entrepreneur, the list of summit participants is a reminder that you can succeed because of your dyslexia, not in spite of it.

Dyslexics search for role models, and Robyn Curnow is not an exception. She points to Winston Churchill who, many advocates believe, had dyslexia; she points out that he dictated, rather than wrote, his speeches and books. "He would have found many of today's voice-to-text tools helpful. Microsoft's learning tools also have incredible options for dyslexics, such as tools which read out text, break up syllables and increase spaces between lines and letters," she says.[11]

Role models like those above and those portrayed in this book are vital, Robyn Curnow believes. In her youth, she had few, but now tries to be one. "Ironically, dyslexia has helped me to communicate to the world," she says.

"By understanding how my mind works, I now realize that my greatest weakness is also my greatest strength."

One of her favorite closers: "Just don't expect us to ever learn how to spell 'dyslexic' (Thanks, spellcheck)," she laughs.

Chapter 7

Gabrielle Emanuel

"'Dyslexia is not something you grow out of. So while I have learned to work with and to work around it, I still notice its presence' in all aspects of someone that is dyslexic. This awareness is something you grow to accept and it becomes your fabric."—Gabrielle Emanuel

Gabrielle Emanuel began her broadcasting career through a fellowship with NPR (National Public Radio) before going on to report on educational issues for NPR. Currently, she works for WGBH Radio in Boston, one of public radio's flagship stations.

When she was in kindergarten, one of Gabrielle Emanuel's first memories was "I would leave class to work in a little closet with a space heater and a reading specialist."

It was a long journey from that little closet to graduation from one of America's most prestigious schools, Dartmouth College, a Rhodes Scholarship to Oxford University, and a position at NPR, before her current role reporting for NPR to the nation from WGBH Radio in Boston. There, she serves as a voice for those who, as she once did, suffer silently—whatever the reason.

One might imagine that two parents who attended medical school and got their PhDs would be blindsided by having a child with dyslexia. In her childhood, Gabrielle lived in Cambridge, Massachusetts, where her parents went to medical school. New England in general, and Boston in particular, is known as among the most important medical hubs at top universities.

Her mother is of British descent, and she saw in her daughter some parallels to herself. "I recall, as time moved to around the time of kindergarten, my parents realized my speech impediment needed to be addressed," the woman who would go on to acclaim working for NPR remembered. "My parents were incredibly loving and supportive to me from these earliest memories.... [M]y mom recognized some of my struggles early on with identifying milestone achievements in school, which she said paralleled some of her own struggles." Being an undiagnosed dyslexic really helped Gabrielle's mother identify the characteristics in her daughter.

"I now know just how lucky I was that my mother was very quick to determine what the specific problems were. And so, my parents have shepherded me through the whole school system," the now journalist remembers. As is the case with many dyslexics, Gabrielle's speech impediment was severe enough that she needed to work with a speech therapist. There was a lot of working on articulation because she had difficulty saying certain sounds or words correctly. For instance, "run" might come out as "won."

The therapist also addressed language fluency, or having trouble putting words together to express thoughts. It was all part of a process, says Gabrielle. "With this help I know there was lots of repetition which is all part of learning and the advice is always to practice, practice. So those were my earliest memories, which started in kindergarten when I would get pulled out of my classroom."

That was while she was in private school in Boston; next, around the age of nine, came a move to Chicago and the transition to parochial school. "This was a big transition for me," she says, but while there was anxiety about moving, Gabrielle was also looking forward to being with her dad's family. The family of her father, Ezekiel Jonathan "Zeke" Emanuel, is from Chicago, and he became an oncologist and bioethicist. Gabrielle comes from a long line of family members with PhDs, as both her older and younger sisters went to Yale and received scholarships, just as she had.

It's interesting to know that her family has long stood for civil rights and giving back to the community. So, she grew up in a brilliant, loving, and challenging family. It's really no wonder that Gabrielle has such an amazing passion, and it's that passion that drives her to give back and help others less fortunate. Life as a dyslexic child couldn't have gone better, given her strong support system and the resources of loving parents and siblings.

The challenge of moving at a young age would be daunting to some, but Gabrielle had already dealt with several challenges linked to her learning needs. "I initially went to this parochial school and then soon switched to public. And for the record, I wouldn't ever classify myself as a good reader. That was always the case in whichever school I was attending," she laughs.

Chapter 7. Gabrielle Emanuel

Gabrielle was the middle child, and neither sister had dyslexia. It must have been really difficult to live in a household with not only parents who are doctors, but also grandparents who were in the medical field and who no doubt observed that the middle child in the family was slower in learning compared to her sisters. Although, Gabrielle says, "I think my dad probably has elements of dyslexia too, but I don't remember them ever being ashamed of it or anything like that."

"My parents were very willing to talk about it [dyslexia] to anyone, whether it was other parents, to my teachers, it didn't matter who it was." The young girl's confidence was built by knowing her parents never hid her dyslexia. They instead had two critical approaches to their daughter's learning challenges: "One, trying not to let me be embarrassed about it even though I will say I was as a kid [said with nervous laughter], and two, they very effectively made sure I was never made to feel like I was dumb because of it."

Research shows that an important component for dyslexic children is to ensure that nonacademic interests are cultivated, and Gabrielle had plenty of this. "You know I was a little kid, so I wasn't particularly smart. But my parents made me feel smart. Somehow I was secure because they made me feel creative; like a lot of my spelling errors they would talk about how creative they were." Gabrielle feels that they didn't avoid talking about it, nor did they make it seem like a handicap. Instead she believes her parents "did a really good job of it not becoming like a defining thing ... like I was dumb because I have this. They talked to me about how smart I was." These positive repetitive verbal supports are certainly telling and became a vital component of cementing her self-esteem.

Gabrielle was in fourth grade when the family moved to Illinois, and once enrolled in school, she was given a tutor, Melanie Mitra. She was instrumental to the core basics of learning to read for Gabrielle. Melanie recalls, "She hated the remediation portion of our sessions. It's a very time consuming approach and I would teach this in the beginning to get it over with. She was always a hard worker, and an absolute joy to work with, but that didn't end in eighth grade, as we continue to have a very special strong friendship now as adults."

Remediation, the term to which Gabrielle's tutor refers, is also known as Orton-Gillingham, and it is not a method, system, or approach; rather, it's used to instruct in how to read and spell accurately, and since dyslexics lack phonemic awareness, this is what's used to tutor them in reading and writing.[1] It's done through a multisensory, phonics-based approach. Gabrielle lacked phonemic awareness, which

Dyslexia and the Journalist

is why she was unable to learn to read. Melanie taught her the painful repetitive learning approach so she could learn to read, which then *gave her the ability to read to learn.* The bond between teacher and student was essential, lasting, and loving. Both speak highly of each other to this day, testimony to the power of a patient, understanding, and skilled teacher in the life of a dyslexic child.

Dyslexic children take nothing for granted, unlike the rest of us. As Gabrielle puts it, "It's those simple things people take for granted like trying to find a word. I don't break it down. That first three letters, dys—I don't break that into a unit. And then the next ones—I mean I can't even tell you how it's spelled right, so I don't know what the next few letters are." It's basically like looking at a foreign word.

The pride is evident in her teacher's voice and demeanor when discussing her most famous pupil. "It has been many years of knowing Gabrielle, who always kept in touch with me, as we had a special relationship. She interned for free with us at the school, as she is always giving back to others." Over a lifetime, teachers are fortunate to meet a student like Gabrielle. "I gave her recommendations for school and all the while over the years, we would continue to see each other over picnics and flourished with the connection we had. I have now moved from the Walcott School,[2] which is where I taught Gabrielle and later I went to Hyde Park Day School."[3] Of her teacher, Gabrielle says, "She's phenomenal and besides my parents' encouragement, I credit Melanie with everything!" It's endearing to hear how Melanie and Gabrielle speak of each other and have cemented a deep friendship built on trust and feeling safe.

The need for a reading specialist didn't begin and end with Melanie: "I share with people that going through school up until the end of high school I always had a reading specialist who was assigned to help me. Sometimes that would mean being pulled out of whatever it was, such as language arts, and having a one-on-one instruction was critical to my learning." We know that having a reading specialist that can teach this approach is central to one's success in learning how to read, but so is having parents who reinforce reading at home. "For me, my parents spent a lot of time reading with me in the evening. You know, doggedly going over the same book sentence by sentence. I remember my dad had a ruler and we would read line by line with him moving the ruler down the book page. It was tortuous and at the same time my one-on-one time with my parents."

Gabrielle's parents complemented what was daily done in school.

Chapter 7. Gabrielle Emanuel

She adds this didn't end with the end of school. The emphasis on reading would carry over into the summer with all the repetitive work with her tutor and her parents. Gabrielle believes repetition and reinforcement were the two keys: "There are some words that I just see, and I know them. It's like instant recognition. But for people with dyslexia, they have to see it again and again and again. And that's what I did when I was growing up. My parents and my teachers would create index cards—hundreds of them—and we would go through them multiple times every day. And I just memorized them because it didn't come naturally."

During her childhood, she and her parents did a lot of arts and crafts. This often involved extra attention to detailed artwork or paper cutting, sometimes using the concept of a folded circle to make snowflakes. Gabrielle's mother was particularly gifted in crafts and also taught her knitting. Lots of time outdoors in nature and running around is how she spent much of her time, as her parents didn't own a television. "My dad spent a lot of time cooking with me in the kitchen, and I attribute him to cultivating my love for cooking. My parents found what I was good at and encouraged and supported me in exploring them."

There were skills and talents others told her she possessed. "I was told that I was good at poetry, which I'm sure I wasn't," she adds. "Over the years they would put up poems I had done, and artwork that they would display around the house. Even when I was older, they would still have them around, as these were things they were proud of that I had done. So again, dyslexia equaling dumb wasn't a thing."

The young woman who would grow up to be a nationally and internationally known journalist had early aspirations. "At one point I remember wanting to do lighting for theater. I had gone to a great play and felt like the lighting had a critical role in making it great. Now I'm most interested in being a journalist and a writer," she says. Gabrielle also had role models, several of whom were powerful figures in journalism history and pioneering women.

"Growing up, I really admired Ida B. Wells and Nellie Bly," Gabrielle says.[4] The former was an African American investigative journalist who also was an educator, abolitionist, and feminist. Among her notable achievements was leading an anti-lynching campaign in the United States during the 1890s. A civil rights leader, Wells went on to become one of the founders of the National Association for the Advancement of Colored People (NAACP). She fought throughout her life to bring equal treatment for African Americans in our judicial system.

Nellie Bly (her pen name) was also a famous American investigative

Dyslexia and the Journalist

journalist, industrialist, inventor, and charity worker whom the young Gabrielle admired and saw as a role model for journalists.[5] She was a pioneer in the field, being among the first women recognized to have talent on a level with male reporters of her day. She is widely known for an exposé in which she worked undercover to report on a mental institution from within.[6] She took on subjects that most men in the field avoided, whether because they were too dangerous or too difficult, and, as a result, she branded a new form of investigative journalism.[7]

"I was drawn to their gumption, their passion, their courage," Gabrielle recalls. "They were both self-assured women who did what they believed in, even if it wasn't popular or socially acceptable. And they both used writing as a platform for change. A century or more later, we're still benefiting from their sacrifices."

Those who do for others are, in fact, the people who Gabrielle most admires. "Doctor Jim O'Connell has also become a role model for me," she says.[8] "He founded an organization that provides healthcare for homeless people in Boston, and I was lucky enough to work for him. The first thing that struck me about him was that he treats every single person with equal respect. He makes everyone feel dignified and valuable." She also found his leadership ability to be truly impressive. "He is humble and soft-spoken but somehow inspires others to work their hardest and to really commit their energy to what can be thankless tasks," she says. It was an eye-opening experience to be working firsthand with Boston's homeless while she was in college, and that, too, was formative in the person she has become today.

It is no wonder that Gabrielle is captivated with individuals like those above. It is clear from the work she has done, and continues to do, that her role models are ones who guide her to continue to soar and break any obstacles in the path of what she believes needs to be changed. When asked if she was cognizant that she's a role model for young people with dyslexia, her answer was not surprising. "I don't think about that on a daily basis or annual basis at all. I have a couple of times spoken with parents who have kids with dyslexia and seen how stressful, scary, and kind of harrowing the experience is for a parent who is watching their kid struggle."

"A couple of times I have talked with kids, and the thing that I always say is 'you're going through the hardest part right now and it's awful because you're doing so much else as a kid, and you don't need one more thing to have to overcome.' But at least for me it's gotten easier and easier, as it's gone, and whenever I talk to them I think like they just have to make it through, and then they will be able to reap some of the benefits of having worked this hard."

In 2013, Gabrielle experienced one of many milestones in her career: the aforementioned Rhodes Scholarship, allowing her to study at Oxford University. There, she received an advanced degree in comparative social policy, on top of her undergraduate degree from Dartmouth College in history. Something common between her and Richard Engel, of NBC News, profiled in chapter 9, is a thirst for knowledge gained through travel experience. While in college, she not only worked with the homeless in Boston, but also practiced microfinance in India and worked on access to higher education in Uganda. Whether true of all dyslexics, a proclivity to travel and learn about other countries is a thread running through all the high-achieving journalists profiled in this book.

When profiled for the Rhodes Project (the program that led to her Oxford studies), Gabrielle reflected on what her experience in far-off places had taught her.[9] When asked what advice she would give to her sixteen-year-old self, Gabrielle's response was representative of her world view: "I would tell myself to be passionate and to really think about how I want to contribute to the world. Also, you don't have to follow one of the predetermined paths that many of your peers will start marching down; you can make your own path and figure out your own steps and destination. And regularly take a step back to think about what really matters."

Local as well as global issues occupy much of Gabrielle's time as a journalist, but also her mind as a citizen. Rhodes asked, "If you had unlimited resources to devote to any one issue, global or local, what would it be and why?" If given unlimited resources to devote to any one issue, Gabrielle doesn't hesitate to answer. "I would do something to improve the opportunities available to the most disadvantaged kids in our society and across the world." In the United States, one of the wealthiest nations, 42 percent of children that are raised in poverty stay in poverty as adults. And those that make it out don't make it very far. We should be cognizant that this is wholly unacceptable in a place that claims to have equal opportunities, and we should be working to change it. That's one reason why much of her reporting is focused on education, both for WGBH and on the broader platform of NPR.

In 2016, while in Washington, DC, Gabrielle revisited a reading center that she had attended during middle school; it was an hour drive away. She was conducting an interview on NPR with a mom and

Dyslexia and the Journalist

Thomas, a nine-year-old boy. "I saw something familiar—students writing in the air with their finger," Gabrielle recalls. She immediately recognized parallels to what she experienced as a child. Gabrielle has used her own experience with dyslexia to uncover, report, and spread awareness about what we call "the invisible disability." Using facts, data, and personal experiences, her four-part NPR series *Unlocking Dyslexia* has become a resource for those in our nation's schools who are dyslexic (transcripts of this series are contained in this book's appendices, A–C).

As an example, in Part I, titled "Millions Have Dyslexia; Few Understand It," Gabrielle did a first-person approach to raising public awareness of the most common learning disability with which she herself struggled. When interviewing the nine-year-old Thomas at that school in suburban Washington—her old school—she no doubt felt as if she were interviewing a younger version of herself when she was in the fourth grade, having just moved to Chicago.

Gabrielle shares in this report what it is like for Thomas to have dyslexia: "It's hard—like, really hard. It's, like, frustrating that you can't read the simplest word in the world," Thomas says during the interview, with Gabrielle, adding, "and yet, while he's in 4th grade, his comprehension is not of a nine-year-old when listening rather than reading. It stands at that of a thirteen-year-old or a seventh grader, but because he can't read the words and needs exposure to vocabulary and increase understanding, he is given audio books."

Throughout her entire series of reports on dyslexia, Gabrielle shares a common work ethic among young dyslexics, that, in the case of Thomas, although he "might want to quit, he's bright and motivated." In fact, her narration states, "that's part of the definition of dyslexia. It's when an otherwise smart, normal kid has a really hard time reading, even if they have a good education at home and at school." These are really valuable takeaways.

She sees Thomas as representative of so many kids—herself included—with dyslexia. "On one page, he would figure out the word there, and the second page, he would see it, and he would have no idea what it said." The recognition in her own life hit Gabrielle hard. "I remember doing that myself. And in some ways, I still do. Dyslexia is not something you grow out of. So, while I have learned to work with and to work around it, I still notice its presence."

While the arts may be an area of great comfort and joy for Gabrielle and others with dyslexia, written words still present a challenge. "It still takes me a long time to read because I basically read at the same speed

Chapter 7. Gabrielle Emanuel

I read out loud. I listen to a lot of audiobooks and take my time when I have to read." Nevertheless, reading has been integrated into her life, along with the other activities her parents instilled. "So understanding reading is still labored and a slower flow than the path of cooking or the arts, which has always been a joy to do. My parents were really careful to ensure I had lots of social projects."

Gabrielle also believes being dyslexic pushed her in the life and career direction she has pursued, at least partially. "I think one of the things dyslexia was really good at was helping me see that I have certain challenges and with the right support and help I was able to overcome them; that applies across the board. Whoever it is has something that they are working on, and if they have the right supports and encouragement, then they can overcome that, too." Looking back, "I did feel if you tell people that you're dyslexic, they'll think you're dumb or something. I used to keep my dyslexia something of a secret not because I thought I wasn't smart. My parents made sure I didn't feel dumb, as I've stressed, but I was worried other people would think I wasn't smart. Yet there can be a turning point where the embarrassment fades. For me, it came sometime between graduating college and starting my PhD."

> "For people with dyslexia, reading and writing takes a lot of energy and concentration. It's draining like taking a big test. And there's an emotional component, too. Dyslexia isn't just exhausting and frustrating. It's embarrassing."—Gabrielle Emanuel

Gabrielle shares this common statement we hear again and again, the idea that "a lot of people have said there are benefits that come from struggling with dyslexia. They say living outside their comfort zone has made them more humble and less judgmental, more creative and less rigid." Having to find ways around problems that others can easily navigate may be part of that process.

In another part of her dyslexia series, she interviewed Dr. Guinevere Eden, director of the Center for the Study of Learning at Georgetown University. Dr. Eden's studies suggest that the brain wasn't designed to read; however, we can train our brains to read. So, now we know that everyone, not only dyslexics, have to teach the brain not to conflate "b" and "d," and as Gabrielle knows from tutoring, it's something that takes dyslexics longer to learn. Spreading this level of awareness through the news media is not only a public service; it also helps drive public policy.

Dyslexia and the Journalist

> "I think, wow, we are one of the leading school districts in the country and so we're doing a lot very well. And it's just sad that we're doing something really not so well."—Gabrielle Emanuel

One of the most pivotal parts of her *Unlocking Dyslexia* series comes in the third installment, titled "Raising a Child with Dyslexia: 3 Things Parents Can Do." In it, Gabrielle includes a number of quotes that are both dramatic and revealing. Unlocking these telling quotes from this series gives us a window into how destructive parents feel dyslexia is for their children:

> One father told me his home life was ruined. To do homework with his struggling daughter, he says, felt like "You could feel the cloud hover over the kitchen. It was just a nightmare every night." Optimism and determination would inevitably descend into tears and anxiety. The culprit: dyslexia.
>
> Yet another mom—whose son and daughter both have dyslexia—suggests changing the definition of dyslexia: "It was really scary for us. It's no longer a reading problem. It's a life crisis."

Comments like "Mom I'm stupid." and "When my child gets off the bus every day, I dissolve into stress and tears," become representative of the inner strife parents of dyslexic children experience.

Gabrielle shares the three most effective ways to intervene when learning you have a child with dyslexia: (1) Early and intensive reading help; (2) Find something your child is good at (for example, cooking, art, sports, music, etc.), anything that takes skill and is something to be proud of. Having another passion where there is a more direct link between effort and success; and (3) Make a financial plan because the costs of outside testing, specialized tutors, and outside schools is in the tens of thousands. One parent told her, use the college fund now, because if "We invest in the child we have now, college won't be an option if they continue to hate school and reject everything that has to do with reading." These are some of the important facts that Gabrielle shares.

Was the NPR series a labor of love for Gabrielle or one that was assigned to her? "It was not assigned," she says, "although I had worked with that editor and he is a phenomenal editor and ... obviously the conversation had come up regularly because he was always looking at my scripts and he would naturally go to that and he had an interest in education so this fit, and then it actually came about because we periodically talked about it. I have been hesitant because I tend not to do

Chapter 7. Gabrielle Emanuel

journalism where I am part of the story. Almost every other story I've ever done, I try not to put myself in it."

"I think I'm old school. It's become more and more around identity and reporters and things but I really like the separation, however, we talked about it on and off and then I actually knew I was moving jobs and in the conversation, this was one of the last opportunities. Even then I wasn't sure that I would put myself in the story, but it ended up making the most sense."

Gabrielle is aware, she says, of the significant impact the NPR series has had on the national conversation surrounding dyslexia; in fact, at this writing, it's at the top of the Google "trail" when searching for information on the topic. "I remember afterwards the letters that came in were just so kind. And that actually might have been the best part of the whole thing," she recalls. "Besides getting to talk with other people who are dyslexic, which is what I rarely get to do. It's the letters that came afterwards that were so meaningful."

Gabrielle has thought a lot about what she would say to teachers and administrators about identifying kids who may be dyslexic. Putting it in terms of her own success, she sees it this way:

> The key to my success was two things: one is early identification, that my parents knew when I was a very young child that I needed help with this. And the second was, working one-to-one with teachers until I got it. Without that I wouldn't be reading ... let alone working with words for my profession or having a PhD or whatever you want to point to. I wouldn't be able to do those things without the reading specialist or having started really early....
>
> The one thing I remember very clearly from when I did those series of stories for NPR, I was going to talk to the researchers because I had actually been in studies on dyslexia as a younger person, but I hadn't actually seen the results. So when you really do intensive reading work, your brain actually changes, and when they put you in the fMRI before and after, it looks different, like you are able to rewire how your brain is reading by doing the intensive work by someone who is trained in it.

It came as a surprise, even to a journalist whose job often involves being surprised by new knowledge. "It's incredible what you can do when you have the identification, help, and assistance necessary. The thing I saw while doing this reporting with the kids is that actually as soon as they did get the help, their confidence increased and their eagerness and willingness to put in the time and effort increased, and then they also had all the skills of like a good work ethic, humility."

Dyslexia and the Journalist

Remembering when "I was researching the NPR story coming across the fact that people wouldn't use the word [dyslexia] in schools and I had never had that experience personally, it came as quite a shock! I think probably because my parents had used it from the get go and made it safe and accepted."

A diet of fun also plays a role in Gabrielle's life.

> For fun, I can tell you, whenever I have free time, finding something creative to do with my hands is a priority. That could be cooking, furniture building, pottery, or paper cutting. I also love meals, hosting dinners, having friends over, being able to simply sit around a table and have a good conversation. When I lived abroad, I worked at a woodshop in Oxford. I've done woodworking for years, and as soon as I knew I was heading to the United Kingdom I started looking up furniture shops and woodworking studios. I found a great one where I took lessons for two years. It was a great experience. In an environment where we're very much working with our minds, it was great to work with my hands.

This brand of experiential learning was a big part of her education, not simply book learning. "I got to see a whole different side of Oxford—a different community, a different set of people, a different set of ideas and expectations. Town–gown divides have always made me uncomfortable, so I really valued feeling comfortable in some of Oxford's various different worlds. But did you notice, there was no mention of picking up a long book!"

On the family front, "my husband knows I have dyslexia. We often watch and wonder with our little son what his experience, if any, will be. For him, he didn't grow up knowing people who had dyslexia; actually, no, I'm sure he did grow up with people having dyslexia, but I'm sure he didn't realize it. So, for him it was just the adjustment of knowing you're smart but you still have this thing. At the time we got together it wasn't an issue, so he knew what I was already like."

Looking back, Gabrielle reflects on how she started her career in journalism as a Kroc Fellow at NPR, and never had the self-doubt that many may have—mainly, she insists, because she had the support many with dyslexia, sadly, do not. As mentioned, in her journalism career at NPR, she gravitated toward stories with education as the subject. Since going to WGBH, Gabrielle has reported on everything from controversial real estate developments to sea turtles stranded by changing water temperatures.

She is in a select group of people who are selected for a Rhodes scholarship to attend Oxford. According to the Rhodes Trust, only

Chapter 7. Gabrielle Emanuel

thirty-two American university students have been chosen yearly for full scholarship, out of thousands of applicants every year. To date, the Rhodes scholarship remains one of the most competitive in the world; its current acceptance rate stands at 0.7 percent, much lower than Harvard's 5.6 percent acceptance rate for undergraduate students.

Understanding the complexities that Gabrielle initially experienced, and then seeing the supports her family were able to ensure she received academically, socially, and emotionally, secured her ability to display her aptitudes. She was allowed to soar and achieve, garnering one of the most prestigious and unique accomplishments for a dyslexic student. She continues to break barriers, though she doesn't see them as barriers, no doubt due to her mother's initial early detection and her family's support.

Over her career Gabrielle recalls some of the conversations and reactions she's had with coworkers.

> Every place I've worked that conversation has had to happen pretty early on. Because I'm always bringing them things I've written and then reading aloud as I practice the radio version. So the way we make radio is, I'll write up my script and I'll put in different cuts from other people, but I read it and play those cuts of tape and the editor will listen. But I can't read that fluently and my writing has lots of spelling mistakes and typos [laughing] and everything in there, so you see I have to tell them very early on about this and almost always it ends up in a really good helpful conversation and there's always the question what exactly it means, or is … that's always hard to explain.

Over time it could be said "I think that's because there are so many misconceptions. I get of a lot of 'Oh the letters look jumbled up to you,' which is not how I experience it. But, by and large, my editors have been extremely understanding, especially the one at NPR who is the educational editor, and he's the one that I did the dyslexic series with. So it comes up VERY quickly."

She still has concerns about how dyslexic children and adults are perceived.

> One of my main concerns when going into that conversation of what a dyslexic looks like is often that for some people it is synonymous with dumb, different, or not good at whatever you're doing. For me, I try to…. I feel the need to prove myself at the exact same time I tell them that I'm dyslexic … and that hasn't been a problem because I don't think these editors I have worked for have felt that. Radio is particularly suited to this, for me it's because it doesn't matter what my script looks like as soon as I go in front of a microphone and track it, because it's just what it sounds like on the other end. And if every word is misspelled it's okay. So that's perfect for me….

Dyslexia and the Journalist

Often, if I'm working with my husband and he'll look at a script and ask "what are you trying to say here." I'll just say it and he'll be like "Oh of course!" So, the radio feels like a good match in that regard.

To have become a successful journalist with dyslexia, who also was initially challenged with a speech impediment, the full scope of seeing Gabrielle's early dedication to doing the hard work needed to learn reading now makes it strange to think she once had such an early disability. It's actually unthinkable, given the extraordinary accomplishments that few attain. Her work ethic and passion to help those less fortunate and in need of a voice is in line with her civil rights views and love of people. Her journalistic body of work, like that of her earliest role models, Ida B. Wells and Nellie Bly, is groundbreaking. She has set the tone for a generation of young people who need a voice, here and abroad. She continues to be an advocate for those who deserve the educational resources that can come from improved news coverage of America's number one learning disability. Gabrielle Emanuel has not only shown us that it *can* be done; she provides a blueprint for *how* it can be done.

Chapter 8

Jill Wellington

> "If a magic fairy had visited me as a young girl and told me I would be a journalist when I grew up, I would have said, 'No way.' That was the last vocation I could ever imagine for myself."—Jill Wellington, journalist and photographer

Despite her own self-doubts, Jill Wellington went on to become an award-winning television news reporter in a career that spanned eighteen years, including fourteen in television, reporting in radio, writing a weekly humor column for her local newspaper in Michigan, and writing for magazines all over the world. In addition, she is the author of four books—pretty good for a girl who grew up coping with dyslexia.[1]

The middle child of five siblings, Jill became aware of her dyslexia early in elementary school. "When I was in the third to fourth grade, I was having problems and struggled," she says. "When I was in the fifth grade, I failed the standardized test and I was taken to be privately evaluated and it was then that I was diagnosed."[2] Things slowly got better, but reading was the big challenge. Writing, on the other hand, seemed to come naturally—especially storytelling. "I never knew I had writing talent even after I wrote a humorous little story in the fourth grade titled Jimmy and the Frog. My teacher had me read it to the class, and for a fleeting moment, I felt I could write."[3]

The victory was short lived, she recalls. "The feeling quickly melted away as I was overwhelmed with dyslexia, often failing tests despite my understanding of the topic. History was the worst. Those multiple choice tests still haunt me as I remember the words scrambling in front of me. Yet if they had asked, I could have written an eloquent essay about the topic. But nobody ever asked, and I was still struggling in my senior year of high school."

The tension became internalized and externalized. "I clearly remember my government teacher calling me to his desk where he held my failed test. Across the top he had scribbled, 'If you don't pass the

Dyslexia and the Journalist

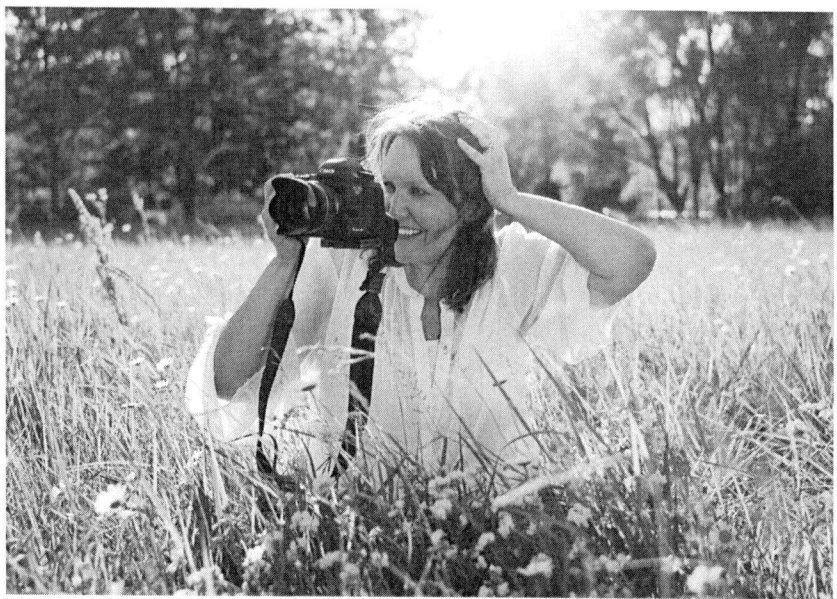

Jill Wellington (courtesy Jill Wellington).

final exam, you will not be able to graduate.' I don't know where I got the courage that bleak moment, but I told him I did not test well, and pleaded for him to let me do a project instead. When this special teacher agreed, he had no idea he was about to change my life forever. I knew at that instant I would get an A in the class."

That was when it hit her. "I'm a visual learner," she exclaims. As with many dyslexics, Jill Wellington had found her path—project-based learning. That "special teacher" took the time to understand, listen, and encourage. "I poked around and learned our school had recently purchased new video equipment for the library, and the librarian was eager to help me create a political campaign on tape. The ideas poured out of me, and I created candidates, campaign platforms, interviews, and debates using my friends as actors," she recalls. It was the first of several life-changing moments.

"I will never forget my pounding heart as I turned out the lights in the classroom and aired my masterpiece. As the lights went back on, there was a hush over the room, then someone clapped. The room erupted into applause and my twelve years of heart-wrenching academic failure evaporated in that moment. I got my A, and the librarian asked if I wanted to create an in-school newscast with the video equipment."

Chapter 8. Jill Wellington

Despite her nervousness, Jill's confidence was building. "I was not a pretty sight on camera with my mouth full of metal braces. Several times the rubber bands would shoot off and hit the camera lens. But every time I went out to cover a school event, I could quickly assess the situation, and the words would easily formulate into a creative, and coherent, story."

Even when the subject was foreign to her, Jill was able to navigate its meaning quickly and coherently. "One day I was covering a wrestling tournament, a topic I knew nothing about," she says. "Yet the story immediately clarified in my mind, and I had fun highlighting some quirky wrestling moves. When I got back to the library to view the tape and write the story, I said out loud, 'I am good at this!' I knew it in my heart, body, mind, and very soul. I had found my life mission." The common denominator shared with other journalists who have dyslexia? "I have the ability to see a chaotic scene and pick out elements and turn it into great storytelling."

Journalism guided her journey from high school to college. After graduation from Sycamore High School in Cincinnati, she entered Ohio University and declared journalism as her major. When asked why she picked journalism, she laughs. "What in the hell are you doing in this, is what I would ask myself." And she wasn't alone. She recalls her brother once telling her she was crazy to pursue news reporting. "That isn't practical," he chanted. "How will you ever get a job in that field?"

But Jill persevered, nonetheless. "I stuck with journalism even though my brother thought I was crazy. Yet I knew he was wrong, and so was the teacher who told me I had a bad voice for broadcasting. I went to the speech department and hired a speech therapist. I knew I was good at broadcast journalism."

"I entered college that fall and still struggled with the classes. But many teachers let me write papers in lieu of a test, and I squeaked through history. In journalism classes, I hit my stride and when we were assigned to provide one story a week for the campus radio news show, I provided one every day. With ease, I gathered and wrote story after story, knowing, 'I'm good at this!'"

Anchoring wasn't her strength, because it involves reading scripts aloud on the screen, but "live shots," where the reporter just speaks to the camera in her/his own words, were. She cites the fact that such reports are "extemporaneous" as one reason why she was especially well suited to conveying them, rather than a set of written words.

She also wasn't about to be discouraged by the occasional teacher who was anything but encouraging. There was "the teacher who told me I had a bad voice for broadcasting. I went to the speech department and hired a speech therapist. I knew I was good at broadcast journalism." And she knew she wanted to do it for a reason, one that went back to her childhood watching television news in her parents' living room.

"The evening newscasts frightened me with their macabre scenes of violence and atrocities," she once wrote. "I would flip off the television if a story came on about abuse or crime. I had an internal instinct of love and peace that didn't settle with what I saw on the news." She was determined to do it better, and she believes she has achieved that goal—and many others—against all odds. " Incredible coincidences or synchronicities guided me through an eighteen-year journalism career filled with fascinating adventures, accolades, and awards," she proudly proclaims.

Eventually, Jill used her visual skills honed in television news to become a portrait photographer. "At fifty-two, my husband gave me a camera and that was my transitional moment into photography," she says. The attraction to photography came at an auspicious time, during a period when she and her husband were in the midst of cultivating an empty nest. "I had no idea why I would need a nice camera with my children gone from the nest. I didn't even take it out of the box for six months. That year, I started writing a blog and realized I needed photos. So I opened the camera box and slowly, painstakingly began to study photography via blog posts and YouTube videos and shooting something every day."[4]

In many ways, it was a great match for her visual style of learning. "Photography is complex to learn, and for the first two years, I mostly shot flowers, landscapes ... nature stuff that was right in front of me. But I had a strong fascination with photographing people. That was an entirely new ball game; to learn how to capture beautiful skin tones and sparkly eyes. Photography is endlessly creative and puzzling.... I still learn every time I shoot. I guess that's what keeps me fascinated!" She specializes "in natural light, location photography. I also create fine art photography that has been used on book covers, album covers, magazine covers, print advertisements, website design, and much more all over the world. Six of my photos were used in the set design for five Hallmark and two Lifetime movies!"[5]

There remains from a childhood spent with dyslexia the need for quiet and solitude to reconnect with her creative side.

Chapter 8. Jill Wellington

Alone time is crucial for me because I pretty much live inside my head. For me, the creative process is constantly waking me up at night and filling my mind with ideas. I know this sounds crazy, but I get visions of the photos before I'm even on the shoot. The visions are so vivid, I see the fine details such as a flower the person is holding or the kind of shoes they will wear. This is amazing and annoying because then I am compelled to find all these props at various thrift stores and garage sales or order on eBay.

Dyslexia has always been a part of her life, even to this day. "I have a son and a daughter. My son is dyslexic, and in the fifth grade he finally learned to read. He was very shy and used to crawl under his bed to hide." Today, Jill Wellington is adamant that no one, child or adult, with dyslexia should be forced to hide. The scars from her own childhood remain, but so does the desire to use her own pain to heal others. In an article she wrote detailing her own experiences with dyslexia, she embraces the healing that took a lifetime, but is now very close. "I have sobbed as I wrote this, revisiting old wounds. I tell this story now for one reason only. So YOU will KNOW. When your heart awakens to your life mission, YOU will KNOW. No situation or person can suppress your true calling. You chose it before you were born, and you will discover it within yourself when the timing is perfect."

Her final message for those who today cope with and navigate their own dyslexia is that all things are possible for those who don't allow others to kill their dreams. "Promise me," she says, "you will not let outward appearances or influences quash your vibrant true self. Everyone has a life mission so important, the world would not be as glittery without you."

Chapter 9

Richard Engel

"I am very happy that I have a mind that can think quickly and problem solve and doesn't like conformity and is a little different from everyone else. [It] is a privilege. Who would want to think like everyone else?"—Richard Engel

Richard Engel is chief foreign correspondent for NBC News, where he reports on all its platforms, including *NBC Nightly News* and the *Today Show*. Before joining NBC in 2008, he covered the start of the 2003 Iraq War for ABC News as a freelance journalist.

Even today Richard Engel finds it hard to believe he once couldn't distinguish right from left, tell time, count money, or even tie his shoes. Engel now traverses the globe, navigating the world's most dangerous hot spots while surviving myriad tests that would be daunting to most of us. One thing the forty-seven-year-old journalist now feels contributed to his survival instinct was having a childhood characterized by all the classic symptoms of dyslexia.

Raised in Manhattan by two parents who worried about their son's dyslexia, Engel knew early on that there was something wrong with his ability to learn like other kids. His father, a financier, and his mother, a businesswoman who ran her own antiques store, also sensed that Richard, unlike his older brother, was struggling in school. That's why, to this day, he remains a staunch advocate not only for early diagnosis of dyslexia, but also an understanding and awareness that it is not an intellectual death sentence.

"This is a really important subject to talk about—dyslexia, but also learning disabilities in general. I actually have a further take on it, I actually like it. It bothered me a lot when I was a kid but now that I'm older I actually see it as a privilege that my mind operates a little differently than the average."[1]

With time has come perspective regarding dyslexia and along with it comes a unique take on what caused him so much trouble as a child.

Chapter 9. Richard Engel

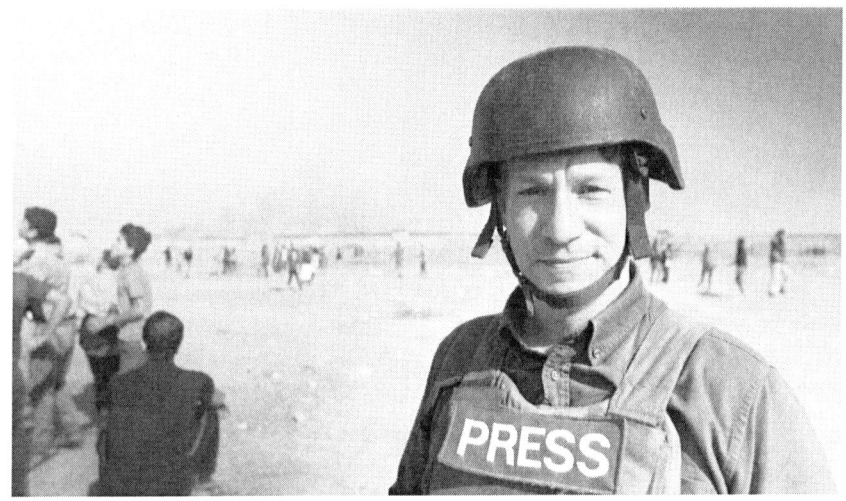

Richard Engel reporting from Gaza, 2019 (courtesy NBC News).

"I like mine. It bothered me a lot as a kid, but now that I'm older, I kind of like it," he says, recounting the nightmare his early schooling had become. "I'm terrible with adding and subtracting. I am terrible at mathematical concepts. I'd sit in class and I'd follow along and follow along, and thought I understood and was really getting it, but then I'd get to the test and it would be just meaningless because the answers didn't correspond to anything. They knew something was wrong—that a lot was being lost between understanding and execution."[2]

It wasn't just math, Richard recalls. "My spelling was atrocious because it seemed like certain words I had never written before ... and writing was just this horrible thing. I went to a Montessori school, and that was partly because of this. So, when I was a very little kid not doing academic work but starting out when you are starting to do more performance-based school ... that's when the problem started to become apparent, that there was something wrong."

That realization hit his parents, who switched their son from the Montessori school in Manhattan to the Riverdale Country School, a private, traditional prep school, also in New York. That's when his dyslexia became more of a problem. In many ways, he began to feel ostracized. "They didn't like me, well, they liked me, I guess, but there were many meetings where they told my parents the school was too hard for me. They told my mother that they should probably find some other kind of school that would be better for me like one for kids with learning

Dyslexia and the Journalist

disabilities." That started a cycle of acting out in class. "I had behavioral problems, I got very frustrated easily. I didn't have very thick skin because I had been performing well in school. I then started becoming more aggressive, short-tempered, I got into physical altercations, fights, lashing out more than once with a teacher. They were not as tolerant as my previous school. I know now, I didn't know then."

He now calls it "the worst period in life for a kid with a learning disability. All the kinds of skills they demanded of you in those early years of school in third through fifth grade were lost on me. Alphabetizing, long division, spelling, writing and writing on the line with capital letters—all those things were things I couldn't do well. I still write with a combination of capital letters and lower case." Today, he says, "nobody cares, but they care when you're in fourth grade, and they care a lot. I was always losing things, forgetting my homework. It seemed like I didn't know how to control my time."

The suggestions started to come from the school's teachers and administrators. "They suggested many times to have me tested for ADHD and have me removed. My mother was in there as she beat a path to the door. But she didn't budge, she said NO, he's there and he's not stupid and it's your school and you accepted him and you're going to deal with him. You're not removing him. So, she was a lion in my corner." Fortunately, Engel points out that he grew up in a privileged household; his father, as previously mentioned, worked on Wall Street, and while his mother ran a business, it didn't take up all her time, so she was more or less a stay-at-home mom. He had every resource he needed, at home as well as in and out of school. "When I was struggling, they had tutors and they did take me to learning specialists, to psychiatrists and psychologists who I hated with a passion. They would give me these dolls to play with and I would throw them up to the ceiling and then I threw them at them. I had to sit down on big plush chair and say, 'I don't want to be here.' I hated it. I loathed it."

All the while, his grades continued in a free fall. "My results were very bizarre. I was in the bottom 6 percent from the computation and in the top 98 or 99 percent for mathematical comprehension, and all of the tests were similar and tiresome." He now recognizes discrepancies between

> understanding and action and execution. And I think it's that yawning gap that made me angry and made me frustrated, that made me thick skinned, because I got things and then I would do a test and the answers were totally incorrect. It didn't even seem like the teacher would go back to it, the answer

Chapter 9. Richard Engel

was so wrong at that stage.... I was diagnosed at that point. I remember my mother pulling me aside and telling me that it's not a big deal, that you're not stupid and she went through a list of well-known people that were dyslexic and this is what you have to do now and it helped.[3]

Still, nothing worked, he says, until he got older. "Once I got older and started writing papers ... once I passed that stage and maturity, that helped as it changed my outlook and performance dramatically and that helped. It was a moment when I effectively got through it and where everything went from D's and F's and incompletes in all my subjects to where in the end, I was almost a straight-A student. And there was a transformation." Ironically, that transformation came not from attending school, but as the result of a small advertisement his mother saw in the back of the *New York Times*. It ultimately became the catalyst for turning around his classroom performance.

My mother was at her wits end of what to do with me.... I wasn't particularly good at sports and I certainly wasn't particularly good at school. Yeah, I was bad at spelling and I was bad at English class and bad at math class and I wasn't a champion at the baseball diamond. I wasn't that either. I didn't have a strong throwing arm, and I was a little bit pudgy. It was not a great period, and my mother didn't know what to do; she found a one-paragraph ad in the back of the *New York Times* for this wilderness survival school in Wyoming. She sent away for more information in the mail, and they sent a VHS tape in the mail, and it was a bunch of cowboys. I remember the tape and it was like, "Howdy, we are the Skinner Brothers," and they were playing baseball—all wearing cowboy hats. It was this wilderness survival camp run by these brothers who had set this up on a nature reserve out in Wyoming.

Thirteen-year-old Richard Engel began to learn things they didn't teach in his school back in Riverdale. "I went out there for one to two months and learned how to tie knots and fish with a rod. And I learned to build a shelter without the proper cutting access and built a tent. And I went on a survival hike for a week-long excursion where they only give you water, and we didn't have much supervision and you had to fend for yourself." For the kid with dyslexia, it was the perfect antidote to being "lost" in a classroom. He found himself. "The way the program worked is the first two weeks were instruction and manual labor, you had to get up in the morning and chop wood before breakfast. Everyone was up at 6 in the morning, and we had work gloves, and I carried a knife around my belt. If you wanted to eat, you had to shoot something."

In contrast to school, Engel says,

Dyslexia and the Journalist

I loved it. I didn't feel coddled. I was out there with these guys saying, "here's a gun and it's loaded." I was thirteen years old and some guy threw me the keys and said, "here move this truck." The consequences were real. It turned out I did really well. I became a natural leader. I started organizing the other kids in my group. I chewed tobacco, had guns. It felt like a bandage had been taken off my eye. This was something that was entirely my own doing. It was amazing and I really liked it. It was a philosophy they had.

For one thing, he felt a major difference between the camp and the school.

I wasn't coddled like I was some kid in a psychologist's office sitting on a plush chair on the upper Westside someplace with some guy with kooky glasses, a whacky psychologist you know feeding me green tea. I was out there with these guys saying, "Okay, here's a gun … it's loaded." Like I said, one time one of the brothers threw me truck keys and said okay, there's the truck and move the truck from here to over there and I was thirteen years old. I didn't know how to drive a truck. It had gears all over and multiple handles and the consequences were very real. And when I went into this survival life, your shelter fell down and you were getting rained and it got cold at night even though it was the summer. It turned out I did really well, and I liked it.

Where whatever organizational and leadership skills he might have possessed were stunted in a classroom, here he flourished.

I started organizing the other kids in my group and I said, "Okay we're going to have different labor groups. You're going to tend the fire." We each got two matches, two lines of rope, a little tiny ration pack, which was something you could hold in the palm of your hand. A little tarp that was like a poncho and a couple of other inconsequential items, one knife and two bullets to the 22-caliber gun that we shared among the group. No counselors, no adults, they would just come in every once and a while and check on you.

It was a self-sufficient lifestyle through which Richard Engel, at a tender young age, learned the practical survival skills that would one day serve him well—let alone save his life more than once—in dangerous war zones around the world. Those skills, he says, made him feel both capable and resourceful.

We give all of our matches to one kid and he's the fire guy, and you guys are going to do the wood collecting patrol, and I'm going to work on shelters, and this person gets the gun and everyone their bullets, and you are going to go out and hunt whatever you can like squirrels, badgers and whatever was out there. We ate steak, birds, and lots of fish. Mostly we ate a lot of fish. Basically, you throw a rod in and you pull out a fish. So we ate a lot of fish. I loved it…. I just loved it!

Chapter 9. Richard Engel

So, when the two months were up and he returned to New York and school, he was a different person. "When I came back to my preppy New York school, I felt so confident. School became a joke." For one thing, he thought about how much he had experienced in life that none of his classmates could even envision. "I had chewed tobacco, lit fires, and had guns, and I thought 'who are all you wussies,' and I felt so confident that it reflected on everything. I lost a little weight and that boosted my confidence." By the time he returned to school, dyslexia aside, he was a new person.

> Here I was at fourteen, fifteen, I had come into my own and I was handsome, and girls started liking me, I had much more confidence. So, those tests that I had previously struggled with, that I had put meaningless answers on, were suddenly ridiculously easy, and I remember going in to test and I didn't even have to study.... School became easy. I didn't ever do well on standardized tests. SATs, I didn't ace any standardized test. I think I did better with them going through this transformation than beforehand.... The dyslexia was still there, but the lack of self-esteem and anger were gone.... I think it was all because of the social and physical confidence and it was something entirely of my own doing. It wasn't something that my parents put me into a situation that I was destined to thrive. There were real consequences. If I had screwed up, I was going to be cold. If I gave the gun to the wrong person—I was going to get shot, or something bad was going to happen. If the fire had gone out we would be eating raw trout, which would not be a great thing.

He calls his mother "the hero here." Not only did she find the camp in the first place, by happenstance finding the ad for it in the *Times*, but she encouraged him to stay connected to it, even after returning home to New York. "After I came back from the camp, I went back for five more years. I went back for three more as a camper and then two more as an instructor. I became quite proficient at teaching survival skills. That wasn't academic, but rather hunting and gathering for sustenance. I'm not a hunter; I don't go out and shoot deer. I don't like hunting, it's not my thing, but it was just a survival thing." Like Anderson Cooper, as a young man Richard Engel gravitated toward the survival skills learned in the wilderness. "The consequences were real. It was excellent preparation for what I do today," he believes.

For one, it gave him a great advantage in his eventual chosen career as a war correspondent. It's similar, he says, to being thrown into survival mode, "like being dropped in Iraq to report and only having been given two weeks of instructional training (like a marine before a mission,

Dyslexia and the Journalist

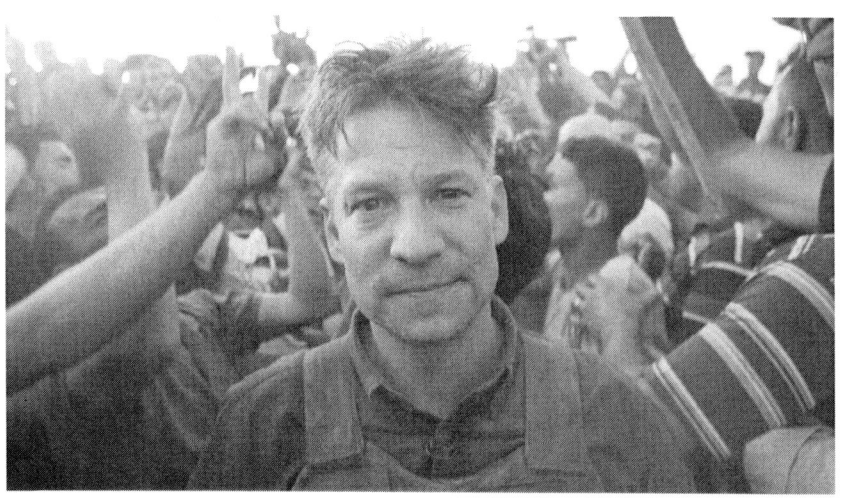

Richard Engel in Gaza, reporting from a crowd, 2018 (courtesy NBC News).

which never truly prepares you) and having had a long standing ability to be able to take charge of a previous situation." What he had developed was the ability to lasso in whatever issue presented itself and navigate and handle it methodically.

That was still a long way in the future, and in the meantime, his parents worried about what would become of their dyslexic son in terms of finding a career. "They were concerned. My dad, Peter, was a stockbroker on Wall Street at Goldman Sachs and didn't think I was suited for that. They didn't know what to do with me. At one stage they thought maybe I would have a business in restaurants because I liked food. They were thinking of how they were going to set me up with some sort of career that I would be able to manage."

The wilderness camp was only the beginning of a major change in his young life.

> I think I washed the funk off of the learning disabilities with the transformation in learning survival skills. I then did a year abroad in high school, which was probably the most transformative thing after that. I did a full academic year in Italy. It turned out to be about a year in Palermo, Sicily. I did a year in the American Field Service (AFS), and that was my junior year in high school. Again, it was phenomenal because I was told I would never learn another language and yet I learned Italian easily. Within two months, I was speaking Italian.

It was just the beginning.

Chapter 9. Richard Engel

When I came home, I had a terrible kind of dirty little mustache, I was wearing silk shirts, I had a motorcycle, and I was dating an Italian girl. And I came back and it was another kind of experience where I was thrown into a situation that was unfamiliar to me, where I was told I was going to fail. I ended up becoming the representative for the program [AFS]. I was one of the students that was selected by the administration to go around to other parts of the country and visit other students as they were having problems because I had proven myself and I had become a peer mentor for other students. It was because I had integrated so well.

It became a deep and lasting experience that shaped his future career aspirations in a way even his parents didn't at first fathom. The Italian adventure stuck with him and provided a lifetime connection to other nations and cultures. "Actually, this Christmas I am going back to Sicily, and I'm going to have Christmas with the same family. All of this annoying stuff, the school skills that I had been struggling with so badly, was irrelevant. Because the most important thing if you are in a foreign environment is that you can speak, read, and write the foreign language, and that came very easily to me because I was social, I liked interacting with people. It was a lot of fun."

The idea that there are teachers who tell dyslexic students that they shouldn't be taking a foreign language, because they haven't even learned English, makes Richard Engel bristle. "They are totally wrong. Nonsense," he insists. "To me, learning a language is like listening to music. It's nothing like reading and writing. You don't see the words written, you hear them. You learn from your parents; you mimic them. Learning a language at any age, you don't hear the words broken up. Then you learn backwards; then you learn how this language that you hear matches the written word." For example, he says, "now I speak Arabic, I speak almost all the dialects of Arabic, I speak Spanish, I can translate between French and Arabic. I don't even speak French. I have no fear of language whatsoever."

That interest and facility with language combined with his burgeoning love of travel, which he had been privileged to experience due to his parents' comfortable finances. "My father used to travel and took us all to Morocco one year. It was the first time I had ever really been exposed to international news." It fueled Engel's earliest interest in journalism as a career. "I remember the hotel where we were staying, which is this grand old hotel where Winston Churchill used to stay, and he'd paint in the back garden. We stayed there with the uniformed doorman, and each day there was news on the radio about art exhibits in Paris, jewel heists, Vienna, and some political uprising in Africa, and all these items I was finding myself very curious about."

One night, the Engel family was going out to dinner when his mother saw Richard reading the newspaper. "She said, 'What are you doing?'" His mother had seen the interest in her son's eyes. "She said, I could see you working there one day. It sounded very romantic and intriguing to me, living in Paris. Then when I got older the idea still lingered there, and then when I got to live in Italy, that solidified it even more, and I had this very romantic notion that I would be living in Paris and wearing a crumpled suit and smoking cigarettes with a hat and writing my stories out on an electric typewriter and writing about intrigue, and I thought it would be very fun, that lifestyle and that mission."

The dream stuck with him while still in high school. "And then when I was in college, I thought *I'm going to do this, I'm going to make this happen.*" Paris, however, didn't seem to be the most opportune place. "Had it been 1940, Paris would have been, but it was 1996, and I was looking at the map and looking at the world and trying to figure out the best place for a journalist to go. Had it been 1986, I would have gone to Moscow, Berlin, or Poland—but the Cold War was over, and I thought the Middle East was going to be the story that was going to define my generation, and decided to move out to the Middle East."

He felt confident making the move. "I had already been very comfortable through two experiences. So, I just took two suitcases and $2,000 in cash, and I moved out to Cairo—without knowing any contacts or having place to live. I started learning Arabic, a little bit in the classes, but then just mostly on the street, in the coffee shops, and by talking to people." He also put the social skills he had learned to work.

> Like Italy or like Sicily, Egypt is a very easy place where it's very easy to socialize. I was an outsider living in a poor neighborhood. If you are an outsider living in a poor neighborhood, people come up to you and want to talk. It is not like London or New York, where you could sit there all day long and nobody will ever talk to you. You couldn't sit in the poor neighborhood in Cairo and not have someone come and talk to you; they would come to sit down within five minutes and ask who you are, what do you want to do, and are you here for a business opportunity.

He found that the people there were just curious mirroring his own curiosity as a journalist. As with many places from which he has reported, Engel felt a common humanity with the local people around him. "If you live in a poor neighborhood like I did, you complained about the things

Chapter 9. Richard Engel

like the elevator and things always break, things don't work, the stairs don't work, the stairs are broken, the elevator didn't reach my top floor, there's no water, there's no window, and the cardboard fell out. And so, you are constantly interacting with people and in a way that was easy to learn the language. Then I started writing for a local newspaper and then the journey began."

The now NBC correspondent is humble about his accomplishments since—the network's chief foreign correspondent since 2008 and, before then, its Middle East correspondent and Beirut bureau chief. Even before, in 2003, as a freelance journalist, he covered the start of the Iraq War for ABC News from Baghdad. In addition, he has covered the Syrian Civil War, the war in Afghanistan, and the Arab Spring. He once described his affinity for journalism as "the prospect of learning about new subjects and having the privilege of riding the train of history rather than watching it pass." Today, he even seems surprised by his success in the field. "I wasn't very good at a lot of things, but I found this one thing by accident because of my mother," he laughs.

While some people may think journalism is an odd profession for someone with dyslexia, Engel disagrees.

> I think for a dyslexic it's a great profession. I think it's totally intuitive. What I do, particularly as a foreign correspondent, is that I do two things: I go into unfamiliar situations and I have to sort things out on my own. Let's say I'm landing in Cairo and there's a revolution underway. What's going to happen next? There's violence, etc. How's it going to pan out? I'm in a situation where I have to understand quickly, figure out the logistics, piece it together, pick out the words among the stream of noise. The problem solving is one, figuring it out and making others understand it is what journalists do.

Again, he makes the comparison to learning another language. "It's like learning a foreign language for the first time; it's chaos." Problem solving, he says, is something all dyslexics become good at, by necessity. They are used, he says, to throwing or being thrown into an unfamiliar situation and having to make sense of it. "It's a perfect type of job in that it doesn't have a huge structure; it's not like a corporate environment or a school structured environment in which there are certain expectations every day. You have to kind of figure it out, adapt, react, and figure out what's important … hear that frame around the chaos and grab on to it and bang it out and put it on TV and move onto the next one." Journalism works for him, he says, because he often is alone in the war zones where his stories take place and adds, "I don't do well with corporate structure and conformity and authoritative figures. I am much more of a hunter gatherer. I just go out and gather nuts and berries among the political chaos."

Journalism also pushed him out of his own comfort zone, which he believes is important for anyone with a disability, including dyslexics. "Had I not had my mother that pushed me out of my comfort zone … had I stayed in Manhattan in this prep school world where everyone was coddled and tutored, I would have been frustrated and I would have been really angry," he reflects. "I'm pretty sure I would have gotten into drugs. I would have been a total failure. I'm pretty sure I would have gone to some pretty mediocre schools where you end up just drinking and smoking weed all day."[4]

Dyslexia, once a challenge to overcome, has become the grace that saved him.

> It's hard to know how to give other journalists advice on how to do a better job, because I'm happy I have this issue. I have that boost of confidence, and it was reinforced a couple of times, and now I am very happy that I have a mind that can think quickly and problem solve and the fact my mind is a little different from everyone else is a privilege. Who would want to think like everyone else? It's a privilege to think differently from other people, and I think it's a gift, but it's a gift that if you don't understand it, it can overwhelm you.[5]

He has some powerful advice for parents who feel that coping with a dyslexic child can be overwhelming. "It's mostly about the parents. It's that turning point where you hit puberty and you start making decisions for yourself, taking the training wheels off, letting you find something, and you can always find something and be proud of your accomplishment." And, he says, there is no one solution, no one-size-fits-all approach to raising a dyslexic child: "I don't like the idea that every kid who plays baseball gets a medal. The point is that for parents it's about if they want to protect their kids and their kid is struggling in some way, it is a counterintuitive thing to set them up in a situation where there are real consequences, but it also gives the real potential for them to thrive, because if they do thrive they can pull themselves out of the dog hole."

Richard Engel is painfully aware that many dyslexics, especially as children, want to hide their disability. "I didn't want to be singled out; I didn't like to be embarrassed; asked to walk outside. I had anger and frustration because school was not a happy place because I was not succeeding there. I didn't like going to school. I would do nothing but fail, and they kept calling my mom, and they would complain about me."

With adulthood has also come awareness that coworkers often

Chapter 9. Richard Engel

don't understand dyslexia—either what it is or that someone they know is dyslexic. Fortunately, that hasn't been the case at NBC News. He never has had to have the "conversation," as in "I'm dyslexic." He says it's just known and accepted. There is one joke he shares about colleagues who say "why do you type with your fists"—a reference to all the typos and misspellings in the scripts he writes to ultimately read on air during *NBC Nightly News*, *The Today Show*, or several other NBC media platforms.

"They have gotten used to reading me because there are plenty of typos and spelling, and I still have trouble between 'there' and 'they're.' Maybe because I know I'm not good at this and I really don't care, I'm sometimes cavalier because I don't actually care. I usually don't capitalize, and there are plenty of spelling errors. As long as they get what I'm trying to say, which I'm sure they do, it's okay. I'm sure they have noticed, but it hasn't been an impediment."

Far from being an impediment, Richard Engel now views his dyslexia as an advantage, one that took years to understand and accept, but an advantage, nevertheless. "I don't consider dyslexia as a disability. I think it's just a different kind of brain; it's wiring. And, once you figure it out, it's amazing. I wouldn't change for anything. It makes other families feel less lonely when talking about disabilities. It's not a disability. You can do better."

When he hears the word "disability," it takes on an entirely different meaning for Richard Engel. He and his wife, Mary, have two children. The younger of the two, Henry, has a rare neurological disorder, a variation of Rett syndrome. "We were hoping [Henry] would grow out of it…. Then we realized it was a genetic condition and he's not going to get over it." As a father, he says, *that* is a disability, not dyslexia.[6]

He reiterates often the mantra that dyslexia can be a gift, a privilege, a different, clear lens through which to see life.

And, ultimately, he believes it's up to society to see dyslexics in a different light, removed from the shadows where many live their lives. "They have a car that can go really fast," he says. "It just operates different, but you have to figure out how to drive … it's not a disability. It's the mechanics of the car that is different."

You just need to learn how to drive.

Chapter 10

The Journalist's Role as Change Agent

"When schools produce kids who can't read and spell, then you can't find the 5 percent who are dyslexic."—Tim Odegard, PhD, CALP, Middle Tennessee State University, Tennessee Center for the Study and Treatment of Dyslexia

Emily Hanford has been a journalist for over two decades and, in 2008, was hired by American Public Media (APM) Reports to be its full-time senior education correspondent to exclusively cover education. APM Reports is the documentary and investigative reporting unit of APM. She grew up in Brookline, Massachusetts, in the 1970s and now lives in Maryland. She has always had an interest in how family income generally, and poverty in particular, affect educational opportunities and outcomes. Her work, not only in the area of reporting on dyslexia, but also the science of reading in general, has received national and international acclaim among parents, students, and educators.

It was the middle of an ice storm when Emily Hanford had a revelation. The woman's name was Sarah. She had just had a baby and wanted to tell her story of wanting to become a nurse, but she was being held back by a learning disability. During the interview, Sarah said she thought she had dyslexia. At that point, Emily didn't know anything at all about dyslexia. " I asked Sarah to tell her side of the story, which of course goes back to elementary school where she was put in special ed, and had some horrific stories. It was clear that no one had recognized the clear and profound difficulties she had with reading, and no one gave her the help she needed."[1]

The young woman told her: "It was a horrible experience. One of her teachers tried to cut my bangs once with a pair of scissors because she told me that's the reason I couldn't read." Sarah's parents were from a working-class background, and no one in her family was able

Chapter 10. The Journalist's Role as Change Agent

to recognize it or had the money for resources or to do anything to help her, and so public school was it. "Tragically," says Emily, "public school didn't identify, or deal with it either. Sarah told me the special ed teachers let her get away with doing pretty much nothing in school. Sometimes she graded other kids' math papers because she was good at math."

The school system did her no favors. "Then, at the end of fifth grade, I was suddenly put back in regular classes," she relayed to Emily. But she'd missed out on all those years when other kids were learning the basics of writing. Sarah recognized the loss quickly. "When I got to high school and had to take a foreign language is when I learned my English skills were lacking, because they were talking about verbs, present participles, conjugation and I'm like, 'I don't know what you call any of this stuff.'"

Sarah graduated from high school thinking that was it; she was done with school. Her parents hadn't gone to college. But it didn't take her long to figure out there was very little good work to be had with only a high school diploma. And that's how she ended up in Jill Harris's developmental writing class.

And that's how Emily met the person most responsible for turning Sarah's life around. It's also the point where, as a journalist, Emily Hanford's own story begins. Her interest peaked. "I wondered how many other Sarahs there are out there. I thought there were probably many." At the time, she was doing a story about remedial education in college. "I learned that a very large number of students get to college and are told they aren't ready for college and have to take these so-called remedial classes." Sarah, for example, was aware once she got to college and found out remediation was needed, that her chances of getting a degree were really low. Fortunately for Sarah, her story ends well. Many, if not most, in her situation cannot say the same.

"I recall interviewing Sarah and her former professor, Jill Harris, who taught at a local community college. Jill shared how she awoke from a recent surgery, and there was her former student, Sarah. Jill shared how bright, capable, insightful, and persistent a student Sarah was and how she occupied a unique position among her students; for one, she was driven to wanting to be a nurse. Jill knew that Sarah's grammar and spelling were terrible, but she always saw beyond that."[2] In the course of the story, which became titled "Hard Words" and aired on APM Reports, Sarah recounted that a deciding factor of her graduating was based on her developmental English class—that to pass the class,

Dyslexia and the Journalist

students had to write a final essay. "However, upon the English department's review after reading all the essays, they decided who should pass the class. It was not Sarah, said the department, because of her poor grammar," Emily recalled. "Jill said yes, but look at the thoughts and look at how it's constructed, and look at all of the rest of it. It was her opinion that the system was too quick to label Sarah a failure in that remedial class. So, Professor Harris decided to fight for her and give them another way to assess her, because she just knew she had the ability to succeed, and she convinced the department to let Sarah write another essay. Sarah did and was passed by the department, reluctantly." Jill lost track of Sarah until that surgery years later, when she reappeared and wanted to help her recover from surgery.

By that time, she had realized her dream: she was now a nurse.

It all related back, Emily realized, to the one person who saw that Sarah needed help—and didn't give up on her. "Grateful that Jill was willing to fight for her., Sarah acknowledged, 'I'll never be able to spell. Let's face it. If you're going to hold spelling against me, forget it, I'm in trouble.'" Sarah admitted to Emily that if she had to take the Accuplacer test again, she's sure she'd be right back in developmental English. However, she didn't have to take the test again, and she was able to succeed in college without good grammar and spelling skills. She even graduated with honors, went to nursing school, and got into that master's degree program at Yale.

"What I really wanted to know from Sarah was this," says Emily. "Are her poor spelling and grammar skills ever a problem for her at work? One of the reasons colleges make everyone pass English classes is the assumption that we all need good reading and writing skills and it's something employers demand." Sarah's response: "I feel like the place that I needed it the most was on my resume … when you're trying to sell yourself. That's pretty much it. I mean nurses have their own pages of abbreviations, of Latin abbreviations, things that don't even make sense to most people, and that's the way that doctors communicate, and that's the way that nurses communicate. Learning that medical language was hard, being dyslexic."

She learned ways around it. Like in nursing school, she says she listened really carefully and took lots of notes instead of reading the textbooks. She saw the Accuplacer test and the developmental English class as hoops she had to jump through to prove she was worthy of a college degree.[3] It brought the journalist in Emily back to the central question with which she had begun:

Chapter 10. The Journalist's Role as Change Agent

I started thinking how many Sarahs are out there, and how many Sarahs don't get through. Because what we know from remedial education is that a lot of students are ending up in it, and that's when I started really thinking about equality ... and started thinking HUH ... I wonder if there are a lot of kids that have learning disabilities that aren't being dealt with and identified, and kids are graduating from high school with learning issues that no one has helped them with. So, from there I got broadly interested in learning disabilities, but then very quickly realized that the overwhelming number of people who struggle with learning—struggle with reading.

Emily's work with her documentary and investigative reporting group at American Public Media really reverberated in the education arena when she produced the aforementioned radio documentary titled *Hard Words–Why Aren't Kids Learning to Read?* As any journalist who is interested in reading in general and dyslexia in particular should, Emily has done her homework, mastering the research, along with delving into the science of reading, she and has shared how there are numerous documentaries and articles on the subject—research that has shown "reading doesn't come naturally, and the human brain is not hardwired to read."[4] It is hardwired to learn to speak, but not to read, so kids have to be taught explicitly how to connect letters and words.

What prompted her to decide to tackle early reading?

That's a good question. It started about two and a half years ago, and I was really kind of a blank slate on this topic at this point. I had already been an education reporter for almost a decade, but I had done very little about elementary education. I had done some work on early education, and I got interested in dyslexia in particular. About two and a half years ago, I spent several months working on this documentary about kids who really struggle to read and what is going on for them, and why many of them are having a hard time getting what they need in school.

Among her findings was that

getting their dyslexia identified and getting the help they need is ... a big part of the problem for kids with dyslexia. It is that there is a core instruction problem going on that the kids with dyslexia are often not being identified and given the help they need, because there's not as much of an understanding about how reading works, how skilled reading works, and what happens when kids are having trouble reading. I really discovered through the moms of kids with dyslexia who themselves have gotten really dug into the research to try to figure out what's going on. They are the ones that really clued me in—like we have, we think we have, a core instruction problem here. We think that the way that we're teaching all kids to read is a little off because kids with dyslexia don't need some different, or other kind of

Dyslexia and the Journalist

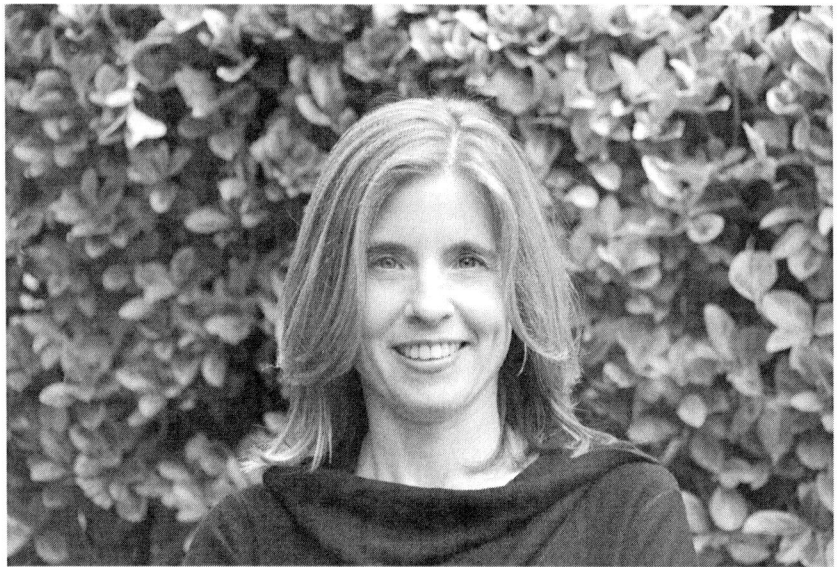

Emily Hanford examined problematic reading instruction for American Public Media in 2019 (courtesy Emily Hanford).

reading instruction from everyone else; they often need more of it and they need it more intensely.

She also realized that "what they need to learn how to read is the same thing that everyone needs to learn how to read, so in some ways dyslexia is sort of treated as kind of like a special ed problem, and really it's not so much for a lot of kids. It's about getting good core instruction. Many of the kids who are being identified with dyslexia may not need that special education if they're getting the right kind of instructions in their classroom." However, her reporting hasn't stopped there. "The other thing I am really interested in is just how people learn, and what cognitive scientists have been figuring out about our brains and how they work, and how that is then translated into teaching and classroom practice ... or not ... as is often the case," she says. "Being interested in those two things at large, I was actually mostly interested in secondary education and preparation for college, and postsecondary education is where most work had been focused on there—the upper grades and on college. If you are interested in opportunity and education and the impact of it, you look at the trajectories through high school and after, and who is getting those opportunities to go to college."

Chapter 10. The Journalist's Role as Change Agent

When putting the two together, her reporting led her to the belief that there is a common denominator between success and reading, as well as between opportunity and success. It became the unifying piece of her stories.

> So by far, the biggest category of learning issues is issues with reading. So, I started getting really interested in dyslexia, and then I just had this very profound insight. I started calling people who specialize in dyslexia like tutors and concentrated on parents. I heard the same story over and over again. I live in Maryland, and at first I was just calling local connections and thought to myself, "My God, Maryland has a problem!" So then I decided to call other states and called a few states around the country and then realized there is something going on here. In fact, it seems to be systemic, and this is not like one screwed up school system or just one state.
>
> For some reason, here's what seems to be happening for a whole lot of kids. They go into kindergarten and mom and dad are noticing that something is not really right ... something is just wrong! This kid doesn't seem to be getting it. The child shies away from reading, doesn't seem to get it. Parents go to the teacher and say something isn't right and not adding up. The teacher responds, "Don't worry about it, he's in kindergarten." You know a lot of times it's a boy because of behavior and crying. Then in first grade it's the same thing, and parents go to the teacher and the teacher responds with "don't worry about it, we just haven't found him the right book yet. We need to motivate him, we need to find him a book he wants to read." The mom is saying, "No.... I don't really think that's it." The teacher says "you need to read books to him," while the mom responds, "I do and have been since he was in my womb. We have tons of books at home ... my husband and I have a PhD, my husband's a doctor...."

It challenged her sense of journalistic inquiry. "Again, I don't understand," she recalls. "Then comes second grade, third grade, fourth grade, and it can get to a very high grade and the kid doesn't like school, and not doing well in anything at school. The child may start having behavior problems or getting really depressed and withdrawn. I can't even tell you how many parents have told me that their little kids who are either eight, nine, ten, or eleven years old want to kill themselves because [they] can't read. When I give the anecdote of these young children wanting to kill themselves—these parents sadly nod their head in agreement." So, she says, that should tell us something about just how critical reading is. "When you can't read, school is just such a difficult experience for you because everything involves reading. It's the way you're accessing so many things, and so you're just behind and confused and give and can't get anywhere because you're 'that kid.'"

Dyslexia and the Journalist

> Oh my god ... think about that ... we have little kids who want to die because they can't read!

"It's interesting to note that since I started getting into learning about dyslexia, I find out that I have friends, neighbors, and family members with dyslexia. But it was not something that I knew, or that was talked about. This is why I got interested in dyslexia, and that was the first piece that I did, and really it was trying to tell this exact story and try to find out what exactly is going on. *Hard to Read—How American Schools Fail Kids with Dyslexia*, was written based on why the kids with dyslexia have such a hard time getting the help they need in school."[5]

The understanding of dyslexia is hard for those who neither are dyslexic nor have children who are dyslexic.

> Growing up for me, reading and writing wasn't hard at all, and I am just one of those kids. We have to flip the script this because the truth is that what the research shows us is that it is actually hard for most people and there is only a small percentage that can learn the way they are teaching. We continue to teach the opposite way, we are assuming that it's going to happen and just click, just sort of naturally occur and there's some small portion of kids who need extra help. It's the opposite. Dr. Jack M. Fletcher, PhD, at the Department of Psychology at the University of Houston, brings up a great point like this quote he shares "We are all born with dyslexia. The difference among us is that some are easy to cure, and others are not." None of us have reading brains when we are born, we have to change our brain, as we are not wired to know how to read.[6]

In the path to covering dyslexia as a journalist, one step leads to the next. "Usually, in the work that I do, I've just generally covered education and one story will lead to another. So I think it's this natural piece that one goes from remedial education, which led me to a piece about dyslexia and that led me to this next piece. I would have never predicted that I would have stuck to this one topic over four years, but this is so important. I generally do not stick this narrowly to one topic, but it is profound what a huge Pandora's box it has been. This problem is hidden in plain sight."

Once you open that "Pandora's box," as Emily Hanford refers to dyslexia, it's hard to ignore reality. One aspect of that reality is that

> with enough of gritting your way through it, eventually a lot of kids do sort of get it. A lot of these ideas are based on there is a group that will get it, and there is a certain truth to that and gritting your way through it, eventually a lot of kids do get it well enough. But one of the things we are not acknowledging in that, is first of all there is a small percentage of people who are

Chapter 10. The Journalist's Role as Change Agent

scored towards dyslexic and it is a continuum. Remember that, it's a continuum in that it continues. There's a portion of people that have a neurodevelopmental difference in terms of the way their brain is processing the sounds and words and some working memory issues, or other associated challenges, and that's a percentage of a small percentage of our people. That's a story from a small to medium size group of people that I don't think we would call dyslexic. Here's where it gets to be an equity issue.

This is where socioeconomic issues enter the conversation.

Think about this for children who have various reasons why they are at risk for schooling not working out for them. If you put a kid who has a lot of other risk factors, in terms of their chances of succeeding in school.... Think of how many children we just lose along the way. All the kids that say this is hard, but it's not because of the school itself that they're in; it's sort of a struggling high poverty school. Or maybe it's because of the family circumstances. Stuff about motivation, even stuff about like whether or not doing well in school is worth it or comes with any rewards ... we are losing a ton of kids, and if we had taught them better earlier where they could have gotten off to a better start in reading [we might not]. Because once you get off to a good start of learning, how to read the words and do the basics of reading, that's the way that you start to accumulate knowledge, vocabulary, and more reading skill, more ability to read.

At one point, Emily's research pointed to available resources. Those who, like several of the journalists profiled in the pages of this book, had access to those resources because their parents had the ability to pay for their dyslexic child to get help, did well and excelled.

Think about it, if you have more resources at your disposal, more reasons for going to school is going to bring you rewards. If you're at a better resourced school with more stuff, you're just more likely to stick out. The other thing that happens, and I would love to analyze this more ... is that when your eight-year-old says to you "I am going to kill myself because I can't read," if you have a way to fix that problem yourself, you will do it. And the way you fix it yourself is by writing checks. If you have money, or you don't have it but have a grandparent or someone that you can borrow the money from or take out a second job—you will! Parents are spending tens of thousands and hundreds of thousands of dollars to fix this problem.

What's her conclusion?

If you are a kid from a low- to moderate-income family, and you're struggling with reading and your public school isn't helping you learn how to do it—what do you do? You have no option. So this is a way that this is so titled in the favor of the wealthy, and it is not just out of disfavor of the poor, but, again, in favor of the privileged. This is not easy, because people mortgage

Dyslexia and the Journalist

their homes, cash in their 401Ks and go into serious debt to fix this problem. Many people can't even do that because they just don't have that kind of capital. For the most part, if you have the time and money you can get your kid to read.

The first of two key things, according to Emily Hanford, is the Matthew effect, otherwise expressed as the rich get richer and the poor get poorer.[7] It's not quite accurate; it's really that the rich get richer and the poor just get a little bit less poor. So the kids that get off to a good start in reading just start going, and it's an exponential curve upward in terms of everything that they are gaining through their initial ability to read the words and connect it to the words they know how to say. Other kids just inch along making small amounts of progress here or there, or if their dyslexia is severe, they make be making no progress at all.

The other determinant is where you live. Maybe

> there's not a specialized private school, there aren't good well-trained tutors where you live. That's a real issue in some parts of this country, or your kid is really severely dyslexic, and they are really going to need a whole lot of specialized help to become decent readers, and they might never become decent readers. There are some people for whom that is true. But the research shows us that we should really be able to, with good instruction and support for kids who are struggling ... have at least 95 percent of the kids reading at least a basic level. Instead we have the majority of kids in this country that can't even do that. They can't even read on a basic level, making them functionally illiterate.

What would be some of the "big ideas" on undergraduate and teacher preparation to help improve how the science of teaching is taught at the university level?

> I'm a journalist and have taken this on where I have a lot of questions ... and my job isn't really to recommend or advocate for anything in particular, so the only thing I can really advocate for is getting to the bottom of what's going on, and I still feel like I am in pursuit of that. That is really tricky, and I don't know that I know the answer, and I don't really think it's my role and that I should as a journalist "recommend" solutions. I could say more only about the things I have discovered and about the questions I have about things that need more investigation.
>
> Do we need more coverage of this issue? Yes. A lot of reporters are going to get interested in this, which is great! I think part of the problem, or the pickle that we are in, that we got in with this has to do with ... and I'm not going to blame the media, but I think that the fact that we had these really big "wars" that we all covered about reading back in the '80s, '90s, and early

Chapter 10. The Journalist's Role as Change Agent

2000s.[8] I think that the sort of terrain or the debate about this issue sort of got cast a certain way, and it was a little bit of a *he said, she said* battle, like there's kind of one side that says this and another side that says that. Then the research started coming out and a lot of the fighting was around phonics, and that has really put us in a bad place ... even for people who for a long time were not accepting of phonics or were against it, or really didn't acknowledge its importance.[9] People like Lucy Calkins, for example, who has had reading and writing programs that didn't have any kinds of phonics or phonological awareness in them at all, yet now sells a phonics program.[10] I think what's happening is now that more and more people start to embrace phonics, schools add a phonics program and show parents that they do direct instruction and we do explicit instruction and we do teach kids phonics.

Emerging through all her reporting on reading and dyslexia is a single theme.

What I would like people to understand about reading is that it's not about whether you teach phonics or not, it's really about whether you understand this vast body of research that's been done for the past fifty years or so that really provides us with this very robust set of findings on what skilled reading is, how it developed, and what's going wrong when kids are struggling to learn to read. Cognitive scientists, psychologists, and linguists took on a lot of those questions and started doing research in them in the '70s and '80s. It really settled a lot of these questions by the early '90s. Then we fought about phonics, and then we had the "reading wars," and then it's been twenty years since then and we had reading first.[11]

Due to the complexity over two difficult subjects—reading and dyslexia—journalists may have become weary about how best to cover the issue *or whether to cover it at all.*

I think a lot of journalists were kind of like, been there ... done that ... that one's too hot, don't want to go there, or the way that was covered there's a lot of different points of view about reading and people fight about it, and there are the different points of view and you make up your mind.... The answer really is in teacher knowledge. A lot of the fights about this stuff involve knowledge and autonomy and why teachers need to have autonomy. The problem is that teachers are not, for the most part, learning how skilled reading works.

So, should we be able to be in a situation where a lot of teachers have autonomy to figure out what the kids in their class need? Yes, if they have a good understanding of reading and how it develops and what's going on when kids struggle. Do kids struggle for different reasons? Absolutely they do. Should teachers be involved to assess that out and figure out what to do about it? Yes, they absolutely should.

Dyslexia and the Journalist

And here's where she sees one of the major stories that journalists often miss: "Right now, for the most part we are not arming teachers with a lot of knowledge. In fact, teachers are being taught things about reading that were debunked by scientists like thirty years ago. The colleges of education haven't got the message. Teachers are going into schools with a combination of being underprepared and wrongly prepared with things that simply aren't true."

Still, as a journalist and as a mother, she has understanding of the difficult job most teachers face—and their motivation to do well by their students.

> I don't think there are any teachers out there that don't want their students to learn how to read. As far as what I think can be done to change this, I would say the most important thing here is teacher knowledge, and I really do think it's important how teachers get invited into this conversation. Because most teachers know that they have kids, and maybe a lot of kids, or in some cases most of the kids in their class in some schools are struggling with reading, and many of those teachers are working their butts off. They are doing everything that they think they should be doing. They are working really hard, and it's not working for a lot of those kids, and they know that. When you start to tell them something about the scientific research on reading, they go "Oh my God.... I didn't know that.... I wish I knew that ... why didn't anyone teach this to me!" Like one teacher said to me, "When I first started learning about the basics of reading, I thought, 'Why did you even let me teach reading without knowing this!' Why did you even let me do this?"

Her research and reporting has taught Emily Hanford, among other things, that

> English is complicated. It is probably the most difficult alphabetic language in the world to learn, which is one of the reasons why all over the English-speaking world we fight about teaching reading: because there is a lot to fight about. For those with dyslexia, the battle is more onerous.... In English, people with dyslexia tend to have two problems. They have problems with accuracy and speed. So they read slowly and they make a lot of mistakes. However, with Italian, for example, it's not as big an issue whether you're accurate. People with dyslexia can read accurately, but they are still slow at it, which tells us that there is this neurological thing that has to do with the processing of keeping the word in your memory, processing the sounds of the language, that's what's difficult. But in English, it's just because our language is complex. It's not like a whacky language, full of exceptions; it's just this fascinating language that's like a melting pot language that has spelling patterns that come from the French, Greeks, Latin, and the Anglo-Saxons and the whacky ways they pronounce things.

Chapter 10. The Journalist's Role as Change Agent

The structure of the English language itself is daunting to dyslexic adults and children.

> So our common words come from Anglo-Saxons, who just had a totally different way of pronouncing a lot of words. So the spelling makes sense if you talk like they did, but we don't talk like they did. For example, why do we spell phone this way, because it's a Greek word, and then you teach that to kids and then it becomes really fascinating…, I have heard from some people who were dyslexic and struggled in the sixth grade or ninth grade and started taking a foreign language, and it was the first time someone explained to them how written language works, and it was like bombs going off! They would say, "Why didn't anyone tell us this before?" And that was a profound insight for them. Another great thing for kids who are dyslexic, although I don't know any research behind this, but is to let them take Latin … because Latin actually really starts to help you understand the structure of English words, and Latin can be amazingly helpful, especially for kids.

As a journalist who has been at the forefront of the battle for reading equality and one who is especially revered by those in the dyslexic community, Emily Hanford takes her unique position and responsibility seriously.

> People write to me a lot that listening to the podcasts and reading the articles has produced a lot of big ah-ha moments for them. That's my goal. I feel like what I'm trying to do as a journalist is to translate some of this scientific research. I think that is what's missing. There has been a misunderstanding or nonunderstanding of what this research says. The headline is that this research says that kids need phonics, and that is not what the research says. I mean the research says phonological awareness and understanding the ways which English spelling works is super important and that good readers have good phonics skills, and good readers do!

She makes a distinction between those who can and those who can't.

> That is how you differentiate between skilled readers and unskilled is that skilled readers have orthographically mapped tens of thousands of words into their memory. How do they do that? They do that through an initial sounding out of words and connecting the pronunciation of the word with a word that they already know and connecting the spelling and the meaning and the pronunciation of that word and that's what scientists have figured out. We don't remember words as images, but we do store them in our mental lexicon as like units that we know immediately on sight. So, as we are reading along and see words that we have seen many times before, those of us who are skilled readers don't sound them all out—we know them instantly on sight. Not because we had five hundred sight words that we are supposed to memorize between K and 2, and that is still how reading is being done in some places.

Dyslexia and the Journalist

She believes the parents of dyslexic children are the ones who are principally moving the needle on improvement of how reading is taught in America.

> They are the ones that taught me. It's really dyslexic parents who taught me this really isn't about dyslexia per say; this is about the fact that there is all this research on reading and that schools don't know it, so our kids are like the canaries in the coal mine. They're the ones that taught me that there is this gigantic body of research on reading. I think one of the problems we have is that this national conversation is being led by parents of dyslexic kids who are successfully pushing for different kinds of legislation and things in school that a lot of that is really, really good, but it ends up meaning that we sort of end up thinking about this problem, I think, in terms of the needs of the dyslexic kids.

Instead, she sees the problem as less specific and more a national problem. "When we look at it through the lens of the struggle with dyslexic kids, you can almost forget about the broader more generalized problem that other kids have. You have a lot of kids that are struggling with reading, and they're not diagnosed dyslexic."

In many ways, she has discovered through her reporting, it's a problem with how reading is taught, but also one of access on multiple layers.

> I have been interviewing some people in schools who have been shocked when I share that they don't have a lot of books, and kids aren't even assigned to read books. It's no wonder that kids get to high school and they don't really like reading. One of the reasons they don't like reading ... and they can read, most of the words ... maybe not all of them, and they are kind of slow, but they don't know what a lot of the words mean and they can't put them all together because they just haven't had a good rigorous education all the way through. We really need to be looking at that part of it.

That's the tip of the proverbial iceberg.

> With the dyslexia movement, I think it is more led by people who are sort of on the affluent side of our society, I'm not saying it's all like rich people, rather it's more of an upper-middle-class movement. I think sometimes those people can take for granted the other side of the equation. A lot of times the access to books was not their kids' problem. The thing that happens, too, is the way our education system is so segregated by income and race. We have a situation in this country where we have schools where you have the majority of kids that are struggling with reading. The kids with dyslexia don't even really get seen.

As Tim Odegard of Middle Tennessee State University said, "When schools produce kids that can't read and spell, then you can't find the five percent who are dyslexic."[12]

Chapter 10. The Journalist's Role as Change Agent

Having processed the research on reading as it applies to dyslexia, she has reached this conclusion:

> The truth is that the reading research shows that the real trouble with dyslexia is that it's maybe somewhere between 12 or 17 percent, and 1 in 5 is too high … the truth is that all of the research that's been done is really converging more around the prevalence of dyslexia as somewhere between 5 and 12 percent, but it's so hard to identify dyslexia if you're not teaching kids to read. The definition of dyslexia is you are struggling with reading in spite of good instruction, so if no one is getting good instruction then no one can actually be dyslexic to be identified because you have to get the good instruction first.

Journalism—and journalists who understand dyslexia and reading difficulty in general—can be part of the solution, even if they can't solve the problem. Unfortunately, shrinking budgets and downsizing of newsrooms has led to the erosion of "specialists" like medical, science, consumer, and, yes, education reporters—especially at local media outlets. Journalists like Emily Hanford are increasingly rare, and that's why her voice is so important. "I know I am really in a unique situation," she says, "where I can read and write about this stuff. I really have tried to connect some dots that really haven't been connected in the mass media before in the same way. I am hoping that that's not only helping to inform teachers, administrators, and policy makers, but also other journalists too."

She is only one voice, but a strong, loud, and vibrant one for reading reform. It's one that reverberates not only for those with dyslexia, but all children and the right to read.

> There are some basic points that need to be made in my work, and I'm trying over and over again in my reporting in papers like the *New York Times*, because getting printed there people do take note of your writing. I really hope my reporting is helping other journalists find a way into this topic, in a way that doesn't repeat the patterns of the past fight, which this is about, like phonics. That never really was the fight, and people still accuse me of reinvigorating the "Reading Wars" and just writing about phonics. That's not what I've been writing, and I keep learning things, and the way I wrote a few years ago is probably a little different now.

It's a long way from that ice storm and that one woman named Sarah who inspired a journalist to inspire others about a cause so just: the right for all children to read. It's a battle that reached beyond one "Sarah" to many "Sarahs." In the process, it galvanized a movement toward reading equality that proved Emily Hanford's instinct correct:

Dyslexia and the Journalist

the problem of one is seldom what it seems; it is usually shared, though sometimes in the shadows. It is, she repeats, "the hidden problem in plain sight." It starts with one, but ultimately needs many, to bring it into the light.

Of her work, its significance, she believes, is neither the definitive word on reading problems in America, nor an antidote to dyslexia. It is a start based on research, not anecdote and science, not ignorance. "I'm hoping that's not only helping to inform teachers and administrators, but also other journalists. I'm trying over and over again in my work to ensure that my reporting is helping other journalists find a way into this topic, which doesn't repeat the patterns and the mistakes of the past."

In the next, and final, chapter we present resources for journalists to do exactly that: find a point of entry into a complex subject, while avoiding the landmines that have plagued coverage of dyslexia in the past.

Chapter 11

Resources for Journalists Covering Dyslexia and Disability

> "I don't suffer from dyslexia. I live with it and work with it. I suffer from the ignorance of people who think they know what I can and cannot do."—Erica Cook, Learning Ally member

Among the many things shared by those profiled in this book is the belief that journalists who report on dyslexia, among other disabilities, are in need of self-education and outside resources before they can create awareness in the public they serve. This chapter, together with the appendices to follow, is an attempt to give journalists what they need to do their jobs better in this important area. Some of what we present here comes from research; other materials include case studies from which important lessons may be extracted. We also provide some examples of "best practices" in covering dyslexia and disability in general. Finally, there is advice from professionals and academics who study the impact of news media coverage on the public's perception of those with a disability.

One of the best places to begin is where much of the most important research on dyslexia originates: the Yale Center for Dyslexia and Creativity.[1] Their website provides a wealth of information, starting with a succinct definition of the condition: "Dyslexia is defined as an unexpected difficulty in learning to read. Dyslexia takes away an individual's ability to read quickly and automatically, and to retrieve spoken words easily, but it does not dampen their creativity and ingenuity." From there the site collates the latest research on dyslexia and contains advice to parents and students, some of it written by students themselves. For a journalist who wants to learn about dyslexia—what it is

Dyslexia and the Journalist

and, as importantly, what it *isn't*—Yale's site is a great point of entry for your learning. Its links to "resources" are especially invaluable for journalists who feel they know little or nothing about dyslexia.

Based on the premise that one can never truly understand someone else's plight until they've experienced it, one especially innovative website creates an opportunity for a nondyslexic to experience what dyslexics see on the written page, demonstrating how difficult it is for one out of five American children and adults to read and write. The page was created by the friend of someone with dyslexia and graphically shows how words and letters jump around quickly in front of a dyslexic's eyes, making them almost impossible, or at the very least difficult, to read.[2]

In Britain, where it's estimated that 6.3 million people have dyslexia (about 10 percent of the population), the learning disability is broadly covered in media. The *Independent*, among Britain's most widely circulated newspapers, justifiably focuses a good deal of coverage on the topic, having even devoted a whole section to it online.[3] Among the stories are those presenting research as well as profiles of those notables in British society who have dyslexia—including Sir Richard Branson. Even the royal family has openly shared that Prince Charles struggled to read, and both of his sons are dyslexic. In addition, Princess Beatrice is dyslexic and as such is interested in charities involved with dyslexia and learning difficulties. In 2007, Her Royal Highness became a global ambassador for Street Child (formally known as Children in Crisis), a charity founded by her mother, Sarah, Duchess of York, in 1993.[4] There are also stories about the role women play in solving the puzzle of dyslexia, which affects more young boys than girls.

Many stories are written *about* dyslexia in today's news media, but specific resources for journalists to learn *how* best to write those stories remain scant. Those that do aren't specific to reporting on dyslexia. If dyslexia is mentioned at all, it is lumped in with other "disabilities," like blindness, deafness, paralysis, Down syndrome, and myriad other conditions. A casual Google search using the key words "writing about dyslexia," "tips for journalists covering dyslexia," and similar phrases, yields advice for reporting on a whole range of disabilities, but none of them direct journalists specifically to the best approaches for covering dyslexia.

It might be argued that dyslexia is a disability that shares commonality with other disabilities, so the best practices that apply to disability would, in general, apply to dyslexia. Yes and no. While there is commonality, dyslexia, as we have seen, is unique in that it has more to do with

Chapter 11. Resources for Journalists

brain "wiring." It is not easily observable, detectable, or discernible in those who have it. Dyslexics, especially early in their lives, either don't know they have dyslexia or hide the fact that they do out of shame and fear. That makes dyslexia different in that it is more an "invisible disability," as we have previously defined and referred to it. That makes it especially challenging for journalists to understand and report on.

Still, there is advice for covering disability that universally applies. Some of it comes from the preeminent school for journalists, the Poynter Institute for Media Studies, starting with the premise that most working journalists have little background knowledge of disability, let alone experience with covering stories on the subject (especially, but not limited to, dyslexia). Poynter suggests "6 tips for covering people with disabilities." The full list is accessible on Poynter's website.[5] Perhaps most applicable are the following, extrapolated to apply specifically to writing about dyslexia.

- When examining how a policy is working, don't forget to look at the full spectrum of disability. Someone who is dyslexic may also have other disabilities that may or may not be related, but could contribute to why an educational or work setting isn't optimal for that person.
- Use people-first language. Be aware of language that carries a negative connotation, for example, "suffers from." There are all kinds of suffering. Don't characterize one person's pain because you don't know it. Avoid sentences like "He heroically overcame his dyslexia" or "She worked hard to beat the disability." Dyslexia isn't overcome. You don't beat it. It can be "eased," "navigated," even "mitigated," but it's **not** "cured."
- Avoid common tropes or stereotypes. Don't turn every dyslexic into a "genius," but also don't fail to recognize that dyslexics may have unique and valuable talents not common in the larger population.
- When communicating in writing with someone who is dyslexic, keep in mind that dyslexics read at a much slower rate than you might (up to ten times slower), and many "scan" rather than read an entire page, so keep it short! Writing in bullet-style is always helpful.

They are also literal thinkers. There are differences in how people think. Nondyslexics have verbal thoughts, meaning they think in words and have a linear process that occurs with a speed of about 150 words

Dyslexia and the Journalist

per minute. When there is no mental picture for a particular word, it causes disorientation for dyslexics.

Because the majority of journalists are not dyslexic (or disabled in other ways, for that matter), it has become necessary, as one observer put it, for others to "become their megaphone, not their voice." In other words, amplify the message, but don't *be* the voice, because it's not *your* story to tell. Tell it through the authentic voices of those who know it best—in this instance, someone who is dyslexic. The freelance journalist Chris Juhn asserts that today's journalists can't abdicate responsibility to cover any disability—dyslexia included—to those with that disability. "It's not like there's a lot people with disabilities who are journalists," he maintains. "And so, if you say, 'Oh, I'm just going to leave the reporting to the people with disabilities,' there's not enough of us out there to really cover all the issues. I think if you do cover us, you got to understand our perspective and not just go on what you think."

The journalist David M. Perry, himself dyslexic, has this insight: "When we tell stories, we have an impact. We should be very thoughtful of what those impacts are: What stories are we telling and why are we telling them? If we are doing human interest stories, which stories are we selecting?" *Representation* is paramount. While a success story of someone who is dyslexic and whose parents have the resources to help ensure that success is an important story, where are the myriad students with dyslexia whose parents lack those resources? What of their success? Are they included? They should be, or it could be argued that the finished story is incomplete because it's not fully representative. As Perry sees it, "It's very important for reporters to be aware of power dynamics, including power dynamics around representation and voice and who is speaking, who gets spoken for, who is an object and who is an agent."

One of the most ambitious—and helpful—resources for journalists who feel they are in beyond their depth when covering any disability is the National Center on Disability and Journalism (NCDJ), housed at Arizona State University. NCDJ has developed a "Disability Language Style Guide."[6] Its stated purpose is to capture and update the language used when covering a range of disabilities. "As language, perceptions and social mores change at a seemingly faster and faster rate, it is becoming increasingly difficult for journalists and other communicators to figure out how to refer to people with disabilities. Even the term 'disability' is no longer universally accepted," NCDJ states on its website. "This style guide ... is intended to help. It covers almost 200 words and terms commonly used when referring to disability, most of which are not covered in the Associated Press style guide."

Under each of the alphabetically listed disabilities, NCDJ offers some brief background defining that disability and makes recommendations for the best language to use when telling your story. Dyslexia is, not surprisingly, among the listings:

> **Background:** Dyslexia is a learning disability characterized by problems identifying speech sounds and learning how to connect them to letters and words, according to the Mayo Clinic. Its chief symptoms include difficulties with spelling, reading, pronunciation of words and processing auditory information. It is a common learning disability among children, although adults with dyslexia often exhibit symptoms as well.
> The term "dyslexic" is used by some organizations as a noun and as an adjective in a non-pejorative way; however, using the word as a noun (describing a person as a "dyslexic") appears to be falling out of use.
> **NCDJ Recommendation:** Refer to someone as having dyslexia only if the information is relevant to the story and if the person has been formally diagnosed by a licensed medical professional. Use people-first language, stating that someone "has dyslexia" rather than referring to him or her as "a dyslexic person." Avoid using "dyslexic" as a noun, as in, "She is a dyslexic."

While the center provides resources for covering a wide range of disabilities, its program manager, Nicole Koester, says that increased recognition of dyslexia's presence in the United States and around the globe may lead to more resources for journalists who seek to cover it in their local communities. "Dyslexia hasn't come up as frequently as other disabilities in terms of the numbers of requests we get from journalists and it really should," Koester says. "Statistically, if we're talking about one in five Americans with it, then it really should be better represented in the media than a vast majority of other disabilities, both visible and not visible … it really is underrepresented."

The need exists to expand the narrative, she adds, to include dyslexia, especially when there are so many disability advocacy groups vying for media attention. "We only have so much bandwidth, shall we say, so groups that are very vocal from other areas of disability, they have a tendency to take up a lot of bandwidth, then maybe others, like the dyslexic community get left on the periphery and really don't get

Dyslexia and the Journalist

the attention they deserve." The NCDJ is a proponent of what Koester calls "let's have more coverage and let's have better coverage." She makes the point that as Americans age, more and more are likely to fall into the category of having one or another form of disability. Removing the stigma from disability—visible or invisible—becomes a larger part of a journalist's role and responsibility.

Dyslexia presents a special set of challenges because the symptoms usually aren't readily visible to the public—or to journalists. "It's really hard to represent invisible disabilities because what do they look like? We don't really know." But she adds that's why seeing through a different lens when approaching those stories is important. "So, now when I make a story selection, when I go into a story or I'm pitching a story, maybe I choose words a little differently, maybe I craft the narrative a little differently because of the conversations you've had with individuals who are willing to share their stories with you about their disability. And I think that's all we can ask for, is to put it on your radar and try to do it a little bit better and eventually we'll make strength and move forward."

Another way for journalists to improve in their understanding of dyslexia is to see stories that are both informative and representative. In recent years, some news organizations have role modeled what coverage of dyslexia can—and should—be, starting with *CBS Sunday Morning*. In 2019, correspondent Susan Spencer reported "Cracking the Code of Dyslexia," a nine-minute segment focusing on both children and adults with dyslexia.[7] What makes it such a good example of reporting on the topic is its emphasis on current research in the field, as well as its point of view: seeing dyslexia through the lens of those who have it. For a broadcast network to spend the amount of time CBS did on dyslexia—and do such an in-depth report that both informs and represents the range of the condition—provides a great example for journalists to follow.

Years earlier, CBS also did a story on a new development that promises to help those with dyslexia read better.[8] The story is told not only in texts, but using graphics, making it accessible both to those in and outside the dyslexic community. That poses the question, do "dyslexia-friendly" fonts really help? The short answer is no. Researchers have studied these typefaces. So far, they haven't found evidence that the fonts help kids or adults read faster and with fewer mistakes. Still, there are reasons some people with dyslexia (and others) like to use these fonts due to the thickness and delineation of some fonts over others.[9]

When producing your stories, be aware of various apps that help

Chapter 11. Resources for Journalists

those with dyslexia understand the stories in which they have the greatest stake. One such app (and there are many others, but, at this writing, it is among the newest) is called Omoguru.[10] Free to users, it allows modification of size, font, and spacing of the text in everything from books to news articles. Knowing how the app works can help journalists, at the very least, be aware of how their stories are consumed by the dyslexic community. It's not a matter of converting the text of your stories, but rather gaining recognition of and appreciation for the audience about whom you are writing.

It is also best to keep in mind that many with dyslexia absorb information through graphics and sometimes even use symbols as shortcuts in their writing (often emojis), so visual material in stories to include dyslexic readers is of great value. While the goal is to create awareness of dyslexia in the nondyslexic community, it is best to keep in mind not to exclude that community itself in your reporting.

In many instances, journalists from the major media organizations set the pace for how—or if—dyslexia is covered. Sarah Gross, an award-winning journalist who has worked for the BBC, as well as CNN, and reported on educational issues, including dyslexia, believes that journalists "follow the leader." If the *New York Times*, for instance, decides to make dyslexia a priority in its educational reporting, so, too, will many smaller media outlets. She believes strongly that if dyslexia awareness is to improve within the general population, there have to be stories that appear in media outside the realm of academic, medical, or educational journals. "I've tried to get the *New York Times* interested on many occasions," she says, "but they seem to think it's a very limited population, contrary to statistics that prove otherwise."[11]

It's useful for journalists, says Gross, to keep in mind that dyslexia isn't solely a disorder of reading, but it also disrupts and complicates life skills. The mother of two dyslexic children, she knows firsthand that dyslexia affects all aspects of life, and she believes journalists should keep this in mind as they approach the subject, citing her own children's inability to rhyme words or tie their own shoelaces as an example of the spectrum along which dyslexia exists.

Dyslexia is a complex issue that, as Gross suggests, encompasses all aspects of life and does not offer simple solutions. Therefore, it often, if allowed, exists outside the realm of how journalists think about stories. She points out that there is a socioeconomic factor in covering dyslexia, which disproportionately impacts people of color, many of whom end up incarcerated. In part, that's due to the anger of being excluded

Dyslexia and the Journalist

from equal treatment in our public schools and, in part, to having dyslexia "lumped in with all other disabilities" and, therefore, undiagnosed or misdiagnosed. The key is for journalists to view dyslexia through the lens of a disorder that has a medical, scientific, socioeconomic, and, to some extent, gender (boys are more likely to be dyslexic than girls) basis.

To that extent, National Public Radio has done an admirable job in covering dyslexia, both from a scientific and a humanistic perspective. Stories in the recent past have both informed and represented the dyslexic community in a manner that brings awareness and enlightenment. One such story, "Personal Stories of Frustration and Success," reported by Maya Linares, puts faces to the topic by showing both sides of the condition—success *and* frustration—thereby giving a balanced approach to the lives of those with dyslexia, reflecting both their differences and similarities to the mainstream population.

One of the best pieces of reporting on dyslexia comes from Gabrielle Emanuel of NPR, the subject of chapter 5. Her series *Unlocking Dyslexia* debuted on NPR in 2016 and creates a personal narrative, shared with those of others with dyslexia, which tempers science with emotional impact. It tells the story of dyslexia using both the voices and the perspectives of those whose daily lives are impacted by it—the most effective way to tell any story, but especially compelling for a topic needing more societal awareness. The transcripts of her series are included in the appendices to this book.

In the previous chapter, we mentioned how Microsoft is among several major international corporations doing outreach to the dyslexic community. Internally, the corporation has also created opportunities for those with dyslexia. Dona Sakar, now a Microsoft executive who began as a software engineer, is a good example of a story in which the main "takeaway" is the range of occupations and professions available to those with dyslexia. Sakar, who was diagnosed as an adult, is the voice of the story, in which she says, "Many people have dyslexia and feel the need to hide it, because they don't want to look incompetent. I feel like I represent others because I feel if I don't understand something, there's probably at least one other person in the room who doesn't understand it." This level of representation is what makes her story compelling—to those with dyslexia, but others as well.[12]

Some of the best reporting on dyslexia is compiled, and often updated, on the Yale Center for Dyslexia and Creativity's website under a link titled "Dyslexia in the News."[13] The same site also includes a "Press

Chapter 11. Resources for Journalists

Kit" for journalists seeking more information about dyslexia as well as contact information for experts in the field.[14]

While not specific to reporting on dyslexia, a vast number of resources are available through the Society of Professional Journalists and its webpage titled "Covering Disability Issues."[15] Its "toolbox" contains information on "Disability sources by topic," "Tips for better sourcing," and "Tips for smarter reporting," in addition to an experts list and a primer on word usage when covering disability and how to filter for biases in your writing about those with a disability.

Journalists can also learn a great deal about reporting on those with dyslexia by viewing examples of excellent reporting on other kinds of disabilities. Here are a few standouts. First, in 2016, *NBC Nightly News* featured a wonderful story about the Broadway play *Spring Awakening*. What made this story different is that the play paired deaf actors with hearing actors, representing the deaf actors as equal to their hearing counterparts in talent and visibility.[16] The wonderful aspect of this story resides in its underlying message: that those society labels "disabled" have many talents that enable them to contribute in a way that is different, but *doesn't make them feel different.*

That's exactly the approach in a story by the reporter Doug Miller for KHOU-TV in Houston. He and his photographer were assigned to cover a story involving disabled individuals participating in a water sports event. The story has become a case study in how best to cover a story involving disability in which the disability—in this instance, being in wheelchair—doesn't create pity or emphasize difference or hardship. "Miller and his photographer could easily have shot some video and … have done a short report focusing on the difficulties of disabled people participating in such an event." Instead, "he and his photographer produced a story that concentrated on the feeling of freedom these individuals experienced while in the water. Most were unable to walk and used wheelchairs for mobility. In the story, they expressed the feelings of elation they experienced during their first time free-floating in the water." Praise for the story focused on how "what could have been a routine story merely showing the event or a potentially negative story detailing the individuals' difficulty in getting around on land became an informative and visual story about inspiration and success."

A 2019 story by the gifted writer Steve Hartman of CBS News featured one of the first Down syndrome couples to get married in America.[17] In a story that Hartman originally reported years earlier, this piece shows how love, caring, loss, consolation, and devotion are universal characteristics shared in common by all communities—the disability community included.

It's not only a heart-warming narrative; it's also good storytelling.

It's important to keep in mind that good storytelling is good journalism and good journalism is empowerment, not exclusively, but especially, when covering dyslexia or any disability. One of the best ways for a journalist who doesn't have dyslexia to tell the story of someone who does is to read the first-person stories of those who *are*. Seek out those stories. Read them. Learn from them. Don't try to duplicate but emulate their style. You can't write them in the first person, if you aren't dyslexic, but you can let your story be *person first*.

As the Society of Professional Journalists advises, "News organizations can improve their coverage of the disabled by considering various reporting alternatives such as first-person narratives, photo essays, and series reporting." Referring specifically to the story about the individuals cited above free-floating, bereft of their wheelchairs, SPJ reminds journalists that "telling the truth in a story is much more than just providing facts. This case is an example of a journalist who took the time to recognize the value of a meaningful and fair portrayal of a group of individuals who don't always receive such media coverage."

There are many good examples if you *look* and many great stories if you take the time to *see*.

Appendix A

"Millions Have Dyslexia, Few Understand It"
by Gabrielle Emanuel
National Public Radio, November 28, 2016

"It's frustrating that you can't read the simplest word in the world."

Thomas Lester grabs a book and opens to a random page. He points to a word: galloping.

"Goll—. G—. Gaa—. Gaa—. G—." He keeps trying. It is as if the rest of the word is in him somewhere, but he can't sound it out.

"I don't.... I quit." He tosses the book and it skids along the table.

Despite stumbling over the simplest words, Thomas—a fourth-grader—is a bright kid. In fact, that's an often-misunderstood part of dyslexia: It's not about lacking comprehension, having a low IQ or being deprived of a good education.

It's about having a really hard time reading.

Dyslexia is the most common learning disability in the United States. It touches the lives of millions of people, including me and Thomas. Just like Thomas, I spent much of my childhood sitting in a little chair across from a reading tutor.

Today, Thomas is working with his tutor in an office building in northwest Washington, D.C. The suite they're in is an oasis of white couches and overstuffed pillows. In the waiting area, a kid is curled up sucking her thumb, and a mom reads a magazine quietly.

In the back of the suite—a Lindamood Bell Reading Center—Thomas fidgets with everything in arm's reach.

"All right, I am going to give you some air-writing words," the tutor says to Thomas, speaking rapidly as if daring Thomas to keep pace. She spells the first one out loud: "C-O-R-T."

With his index finger, Thomas writes the letters sloppily in the air.

Appendix A

Then his tutor asks a question: What sound do the two middle letters make? "Eer? Aar?"

Thomas squints at whatever visual memory he can retain from the letters he has just scribbled in the air. Then, with a burst of enthusiasm, he stumbles on the answer: "Or!"

"Good job!" his tutor replies, with what seems like genuine excitement, before moving on to her next question about the letters.

I also have a question for Thomas: What's it like to have dyslexia?

Thomas stops his fidgeting. "It's hard," he pauses. "Like, really hard."

Thomas, 9, has trouble reading, but he likes books. Just give him the audio version, he says, and he'll "listen to the book on Audible like 10,000 times."

"His comprehension is that of a 13-year-old," says Geva Lester, Thomas' mom. "He can understand Harry Potter, but he can't read it."

Before they started coming to this Lindamood Bell Reading Center, Lester says, she'd watch with alarmed confusion as her son struggled with the most basic text: "See Spot run."

She remembers trying to read with him. "On one page he would figure out the word: 'There.' And on the second page, he would see it and he would have no idea what it said."

Sitting there with Thomas and his mom, I remember doing that myself—and in some ways, I still do.

As a child, my dyslexia was a closely guarded secret. In kindergarten, I'd leave class to work in a tiny closet, with a space heater and a reading specialist. Walking there, down the locker-lined hallways, I'd avoid eye contact, hoping nobody would notice me.

In middle school, I struggled to read even picture books. In class, I'd pretend. Then, at home, I'd listen to my books on cassette tapes—at double speed. And during the summer, I'd go to Lindamood Bell, just like Thomas. (The reading centers, which offer tutoring and reading programs around the world, also provide financial support for NPR.)

Over the years, I survived by memorizing words. It started with boxes and boxes of index cards. I'd practice each night, looking at a word and saying its sound as quickly as I could. I memorized hundreds and hundreds—maybe a few thousand—words this way.

I've never been able to sound out unfamiliar words. And I still can't.

When I come across a word I don't know, I freeze. It's often a last name or a street name that never made it onto those index cards. It takes a great deal of focus for me to clump the letters into groups, link those groups with sounds and, finally, string those sounds together.

"Millions Have Dyslexia, Few Understand It"

Since dyslexia is not something you outgrow, I have learned to work with it, and work around it. It's always there, but it is rarely the focus of my thoughts. That was true through college and graduate school, but when I became an education reporter, it changed.

As I returned to elementary school classrooms and interviewed parents and teachers, dyslexia kept popping up in places I didn't expect. I saw teachers who were mystified by their students' struggles and parents whose stamina and empathy were tested.

Dyslexia is so widespread that it forces schools and parents to take action. And yet, it is deeply misunderstood. Even basic questions don't have easy answers.

Exactly how many people around the world have dyslexia? Well, it's complicated. Estimates vary greatly, partly because it depends on what country or *language you are talking about* (English speakers may be more likely to have it than, say, Italian speakers) and partly because many people who have dyslexia never get a formal diagnosis. However, most estimates in the United States put it at somewhere between 5 and 17 percent of the population. Many people think that dyslexia is seeing letters in the wrong order, or getting b and d mixed up. Not true. Researchers, experts and people with dyslexia dismiss these as common misconceptions.

So, if dyslexia isn't any of those things people think it is, then what is it?

"It's basically like looking at a foreign word," says Jonathan Gohrband. He's a videographer in Chicago and, at 31, he says dyslexia is still part of his daily life.

When reading, Gohrband says, his eyes often lurch to a stop in front of a word that looks utterly unfamiliar. His best solution, he says, is to turn to his girlfriend, asking a now familiar question: "What's this word?" And as she answers, he almost always has the same response: "Of course that's what it is!"

Here's the thing: There's nothing wrong with Jonathan Gohrband's vocabulary. Or 9-year-old Thomas Lester's vocabulary. They know what "galloping" means. And they can use the word in spoken English 20 different ways. They just can't read the word.

That's why dyslexia used to be called "word blindness." People with dyslexia don't naturally process the written word. They don't easily break it into smaller units that can be turned into sounds and stitched together.

This makes reading a laborious—even exhausting—process.

Appendix A

Writing, too. Gohrband remembers when his former boss pulled him aside after she'd received emails littered with spelling mistakes.

"'Hey, I know it's the weekend, but don't email when you're drunk,'" he recalls her saying. He was, of course, perfectly sober—just dyslexic. Now, he can spend hours scouring emails he's drafted, looking for typos. "It's very time-consuming and very exhausting."

Consuming. Exhausting. There's an emotional dimension, too. Gohrband recalls that when he was a child he would fantasize about not "being broken." He would avoid telling people about it: "If they know that you're dyslexic, they'll think you're dumb."

Yet, he says, there came a turning point when the shame faded. For him, it was when he found videography. There he discovered a "language" that came easily, and suddenly his talents were visible to others.

"I felt so much more confident," he says.

And with time, Gohrband says, he has found benefits hidden inside his struggles. He thinks that being pushed outside his comfort zone by dyslexia has made him more creative and less judgmental.

I've felt that myself, and as I've talked with many others, I heard one thing again and again: When things don't come easy, you learn to try new things and work hard at them.

Appendix B

"Raising a Child with Dyslexia: 3 Things Parents Can Do" by Gabrielle Emanuel

National Public Radio, November 29, 2016

A mother who spent years coaching and encouraging her dyslexic son recalls his childhood with one pervasive feeling: "It was really scary."

One father told me his home life was ruined. Trying to do homework with his struggling daughter, he says, felt like "a nightmare every night." Optimism and determination would inevitably descend into tears and anxiety. The culprit: dyslexia.

Yet another mom—whose son and daughter both have dyslexia—suggests changing the definition of dyslexia: "It's no longer a reading problem. It's a life crisis."

As the most common learning disability, dyslexia affects somewhere between 5 and 17 percent of the U.S. population. Its reach extends far beyond the classroom, causing stress, tension and confusion for families with a dyslexic child.

But experts and parents say there are three key things that can help.

1. The sooner you intervene, the better

When Megan Lordos' daughter was a toddler, there were hints.

Canela Jayne loved books, but hated letters. Halfway through reading a story, Lordos would often try to sneak in a quick lesson about which letter makes which sound. But Canela Jayne would have none of it. She'd jump off her mom's lap, effectively ending story time.

There were other hints, too: Canela Jayne hated wearing shirts with words on them. She didn't want to be that close to letters. Rhyming felt like an impossible task for her. And as she entered and progressed in

Appendix B

school, she sat in frustration while her classmates sped ahead with their reading.

When Lordos worried, friends assured her that each child matures at a different pace.

But soon, her daughter began to dread going to school. "There were days when she could not get on the bus," says Lordos.

Sitting at the kitchen table in their Virginia home, Lordos recalls how Canela Jayne would refuse to get out of bed, then refuse to get dressed and, eventually, she'd refuse to get out of the car at school.

Lordos remembers looking at her daughter and seeing "this look of fear in her huge eyes." Then, she says, Canela Jayne would plead: "Mommy, I can't do this. I can't do this. Don't make me do this."

Canela Jayne's school didn't seem worried. Lordos says they kept telling her: "Well, let's wait six more months, and we'll see what happens."

When Canela Jayne was eventually diagnosed with dyslexia, it felt to Lordos like valuable time had slipped away. Experts worry that this happens a lot. The research suggests *early and intensive reading help* is most effective. And many say starting specific reading programs at a young age has been successful.

2. Find something else your child is really good at

With lime green walls and craft projects on every visible surface, Canela Jayne Lordos' bedroom is an artistic 10-year-old's dream.

As light spills in from the backyard, she picks up a little wax figurine she made. This one is a monkey, one of dozens of intricate animals she sculpted using only the red wax that wraps the cheese her parents buy at the grocery store.

"I take one half to make the body," she says, explaining the process carefully. Then, she turns to another favorite activity—embroidery. Here, her explanation is about her motivation: She likes embroidery because it lets her write with pictures—a mode far easier for Canela Jayne than writing with letters.

Besides her bedroom, she tells me, her other favorite room is the kitchen. She loves standing on her stool at the counter, cooking. Scones. Biscotti. Banana bread. She is even willing to read the recipe, if that's necessary.

Although Canela Jayne now spends much of her summer days with tutors at reading centers, her mother has carved out time each year for her daughter to trade books for a spatula and cooking camp. Canela Jayne looks forward to it all year.

"Raising a Child with Dyslexia: 3 Things Parents Can Do"

For other kids, it's sports, computers, music—anything that takes skill and builds confidence and pride.

Experts say that children with dyslexia are at *a higher risk for depression*. And having another passion—where there's a more direct link between effort and success—is helpful.

3. Make a financial plan

Schools are supposed to help children with dyslexia, but many don't have the resources to do so. That means parents who can afford it often bear the cost of outside testing, specialized tutors, reading centers and, of course, private schools.

Some families estimate that they spend upwards of tens of thousands—if not hundreds of thousands—of dollars helping their kids learn to read before high school graduation.

Lordos and her husband say they were faced with what felt like an impossibly hard trade-off: college tuition or reading tutors. Eventually, they decided to "invest in the child that we have now."

"You know," she adds, "college won't be an option if they continue to hate school and reject everything that has to do with reading."

After more than 400 hours of intensive tutoring, Canela Jayne is doing much better. She no longer complains about going to school in the mornings. And, while she's still in the process of learning to read, she's making strides.

The biggest change, Lordos says, it's that her daughter is "much, much happier."

Appendix C

"Dyslexia: The Learning Disability That Must Not Be Named" by Gabrielle Emanuel

National Public Radio, December 3, 2016

Megan Lordos, a middle school teacher, says she was not allowed to use the word "dyslexia."

She's not alone. Parents and teachers across the country have raised concerns about some schools hesitating, or completely refusing, to say the word.

As the most common learning disability in the U.S., dyslexia affects somewhere between 5 and 17 percent of the population. That means millions of school children around the country struggle with it.

Under the Individuals with Disabilities Education Act (IDEA), schools are required to provide special services to help these students—things like reading tutors and books on tape. But those special services can be expensive, and many schools don't have the resources to provide these accommodations.

That has led some parents and advocates to worry that some schools are making a careful calculation: If they don't acknowledge the issue—or don't use the word "dyslexia"—then they are not obligated to provide services.

Last year, when Lordos was teaching English at a public school in Arlington, Virginia, she recalls a parent-teacher meeting in the conference room. Things started smoothly.

Lordos says two parents had come in to talk with teachers and administrators about their son—Lordos' student, an eighth-grader—who was struggling to read.

Partway through the meeting, Lordos says she suggested that the student might have orthographic dyslexia. Two of Lordos' own children

"Dyslexia: The Learning Disability That Must Not Be Named"

have dyslexia and, she says, she noticed her student had similar challenges to the ones she'd seen at home.

"When I mentioned that in the meeting, I was stopped." Lordos remembers being interrupted. "They said: 'Oh no no. We don't say that.'"

It wasn't until after the meeting adjourned and the parents left that Lordos understood why. She says the woman chairing the meeting came over and apologized, explaining why they were not supposed to use the word.

"'We're not allowed to say it because we don't have the capabilities to support that particular learning difference,'" Lordos recalls the school administrator saying.

Long after Megan Lordos left the conference room, that moment and that explanation lingered with her.

"I think: Wow. We are one of the leading school districts in the country. And so, we are doing a lot very well. And it's just sad that we're doing something really not so well."

Several parents in the district recounted similar experiences.

However, Brenda Wilks, an assistant superintendent of the Arlington Public Schools, says educators and administrators there use the term dyslexia, but they have to use it carefully. That's because educators cannot officially diagnose dyslexia.

She says this approach can lead to "unfortunate misunderstandings." To help the situation, the district launched a Dyslexia Task Force last year. Its website now has a page explaining dyslexia, the district has expanded literacy screening, and it has hosted training sessions to inform teachers about the disability.

"Many years ago it wasn't a word that was widely used," says Kelly Krug, who is co-chairing the task force. "And in the past few years, it's really become a focus."

Both Megan Lordos and the other parents say things are beginning to get better. But this issue is not limited to Arlington, and the U.S. Department of Education is paying attention.

"When we received the first letter, we thought it was perhaps an anomaly," says Ruth Ryder, acting director of the department's Office of Special Education Programs.

"But then as we started receiving more and more letters. It became clear it was an issue that we needed to address."

Late last year, the Department of Education wrote a public letter clarifying that there is nothing legally preventing schools from saying the word.

Appendix C

Ryder says they heard from school administrators about what might be going on: "What we were told was that, when they used the term 'dyslexia,' then families thought that it meant they would get a specific kind of instructional program."

IDEA requires schools to help students who have dyslexia—just like any other disability—but the exact help they receive is decided locally. Some kids may get a trained reading specialist, others could get one-on-one tutoring, and still others might receive adaptive technology.

Hal Malchow, of the International Dyslexia Association, says there's another factor at play: money. He says those special services are all things the school district could have to fund.

And since there are so many American school children who have dyslexia, that price tag adds up—and school budgets are tight.

"Schools engage in strategies to lower their special education expenses," says Malchow. "And dyslexia is by far the largest group within the special education category."

But, he says: "not addressing reading problems could cost a lot more in the long run."

Appendix D
Recognizing If Your Child Is Dyslexic

Do you recognize any of these signs and symptoms below?

- Poor penmanship. All students benefit and should be using cursive.
- Student seems more intelligent than his/her reading.
- Reading is very slow and hesitant.
- Often substitutes words with the same meaning for words in text that they can't pronounce such as "car" for "automobile."
- Misses small connecting sight words like "the," "on," "an."
- Reverses letters like "b" for "d," "p" for "q," etc.
- Turns letters upside down like "n" for "u," "m" for "w," etc.
- Reverses or misreads numbers like "6" for "9," "3" for "5," etc.
- Reads letters or numbers in the wrong order like "left" for "felt," "chidl" for "child," "act" for "cat," "423" for "234," etc.
- Reads some words in reverse like "on" for "no," "was" for "saw," etc.
- Difficulty in breaking down unfamiliar words into letter-sound segments and will omit parts of words when reading.
- Difficulty with rhyming.
- May be late bloomer with talking or baby talk like "pasgetti," "stupermaket," etc.
- May be, or have been late, in walking or may not be coordinated.
- May have difficulty with short-term memory.
- Requires extra time and effort to read and process language information.
- Hallmark characteristic of dyslexia is a breakdown in phoneme awareness.

(Source for above: Yale University—Child Mind Institute)

Appendix D

Other common challenges include:

* Tying shoes
* Telling analogue time
* Counting money
* Mastering multiplication tables
* Sensory issues (sound, touch, taste, etc.)

According to the Yale study, girls are diagnosed less with dyslexia, perhaps due to the manner in which boys express their frustration in an outwardly directed fashion, in contrast to girls who, some research suggests, tend to internalize their feelings and not draw undue attention to themselves in class. Other research suggests that girls tend to process language neurologically in a more sophisticated manner than do boys.

Appendix E
Fun Facts About Dyslexia

- If approximately 20 percent of children in school have learning disabilities, the percentage of that 20 percent having dyslexia is approximately 80 percent, because it is the most common learning disability, affecting one in five children.
- 50 percent of dyslexics are left handed. Only 11 percent of the total population is left handed.
- The word dyslexia comes from two Greek words: dys, which means difficulty, and lexis, which refers to language or words.
- Those with dyslexia use only the right side of the brain to process language, while nondyslexics use three areas on the left side of the brain to process language.
- Children do not outgrow dyslexia, and it isn't "cured"—rather one develops coping skills.
- Dyslexia is hereditary and is on a spectrum from mild to severe. It is said that if one parent has it, you have a 50 percent chance of inheriting it, and if both parents are dyslexic, it would be 100 percent.
- Did you know that 25 percent of CEOs are dyslexic, but many don't want to talk about it?
- On September 18, 2014, the U.S. House of Representatives Committee on Science, Space, and Technology held hearings on "The Science of Dyslexia," a historic first.
- The United Kingdom recruits agents and specifically seeks out those with dyslexia because of their lateral thinking.
- Many dyslexics possess a better sense of spatial relationships and better usage of the right brain.
- Many others possess excellent conceptualization skills, reasoning, imagination, and the ability to grasp abstractions.

Appendix E

    Therefore it is often said that dyslexics possess a strong ability to see concepts from a "big picture perspective."
- Dyslexic people tend to be more curious, a "Why Child," and are often more creative and intuitive than the average person.

One thing I was surprised to learn: you can be blind or deaf and also be dyslexic. Once dyslexic, you are always dyslexic due to the hardwiring of the brain. It's neurological in origin, and it never goes away. It is not a disease, and in the end you should know that without the proper support and education in the science of reading, children will be left to feel self-conscious and inadequate. We soon learn we are different from the kids in our class who all seem to "get it."—Suzanne Arena, "Decoding Dyslexia, Rhode Island"

Appendix F
Famous Dyslexics in History

- F. Scott Fitzgerald, best known for his novel *The Great Gatsby*, was one of the greatest American writers of the twentieth century and is believed to have had dyslexia. He was kicked out of school at twelve for not paying attention and yet went on to succeed as a writer.
- Agatha Christie is the best-selling author of all time, but she couldn't balance her own checkbook because of her learning disability, which was never diagnosed but believed to be dysgraphia. She was an "extraordinarily bad speller" and poor at remembering numbers—but she never allowed her disability to hold her back.
- Scott Adams, the creator of the comic strip *Dilbert*, diagnosed himself, as many others do.
- Dav Pilkey, who wrote and illustrated the Captain Underpants book series, was fortunate to be diagnosed with ADHD and dyslexia at an early age.
- Henry Winkler starred in the TV series *Happy Days* and co-authored the popular Hak Zipzer children's book series. He was diagnosed at thirty-one.
- Patricia Polacco, children's book author and illustrator, is a prolific writer. She was unable to read until fourteen and suffered with severe undiagnosed dyslexia until her teacher recognized her disability. Throughout her more than 114 books, she shares stories about her disability.
- Richard Ford is a Pulitzer Prize–winning American author and a dyslexic. He loved literature and believes dyslexia actually helped him become a better reader because he had to slow down and pore over sentences, receptive not just to the

Appendix F

cognitive aspect of sentences but also to the "poetical" aspects of language.

➤ The author Octavia Butler was one of the few African American women in American science fiction. She was the first science fiction writer to receive a MacArthur Foundation Genius Grant. She was a diagnosed dyslexic and started writing stories at ten years old, as she loved to daydream. Although very shy, she lost herself in her books and writing her own.

Among other recognizable individuals with dyslexia are Sir Richard Branson, founder and CEO of Virgin Airlines; the comedians Whoopi Goldberg and Jay Leno; the actresses Jennifer Aniston and Kyra Sedgwick; and the singer Cher.

Appendix G

"5 Reasons Why Dyslexics Make Great Communicators" by Kate Griggs, Founder/CEO, Made By Dyslexia

Here's a fact: 9 out of 10 dyslexics have poor spelling, punctuation and grammar, but many are amazing communicators.

From Pulitzer Prize–winning journalists to respected CNN news anchors, high-profile Bishops to gifted space communicators, dyslexics use their curiosity and passion to explore the world, understand complex situations or facts and explain them to others in a way that's simple and easy to understand.

So why do dyslexics make such good communicators?

Here are 5 reasons:

1. Dyslexics make sense of the bigger picture.

The dyslexic brain is wired differently, so we are able to connect stories and see patterns in narratives where others may not. This makes us adept at understanding big ideas or evolving situations and explaining them to others.

Many of us become skilled journalists and TV presenters, helping our audience to make sense of world events and situations which are constantly changing. CNN news anchors Robyn Curnow and Anderson Cooper are both made by dyslexia.

Robyn Curnow says:

> Generally, TV news is an amazing place to trust your dyslexic instincts. You have to look at the big picture, identify the story, tell the story and create a narrative that's simplified, so that an audience can understand the main issues.

Like 4 out of 5 people, Robyn Curnow attributes her success to her dyslexic strengths. She says:

Appendix G

> To write for television news is like a dyslexic dream ... the sentences are simple, you're writing to pictures and you need to take away all the useless information. It has to be the real essence of the story.

Her ability to quickly summarize a situation, or assess the facts and present an angle, comes as a result of her dyslexic communication skills.

Thinking about his role as a story teller, CNN news anchor Anderson Cooper says:

> A lot of compelling stories in the world aren't being told, and the fact that people don't know about them compounds the suffering.

2. Dyslexics are great at simplifying.

Dyslexic minds are great at stripping away unnecessary detail to create clear, compelling messages. This means they excel in careers where explaining, educating or influencing are key, like: teaching, marketing, journalism, campaigning or public relations.

Roland Rudd, founder and chairman of the PR firm Finsbury, explains:

> Being dyslexic enables you to simplify things very quickly. It enabled me to see the big picture and I could make decisions more creatively and effectively as a result.

Other dyslexic minds, like the space scientist and communicator Maggie Aderin-Pocock, use their dyslexic communication skills to simplify concepts that are "out of this world" and go on to engage new audiences and inspire a generation.

"As a scientist, I have found that I am able to take complex ideas and simplify them, story tell and bring science ideas to life in my own unique way, this has been a huge advantage," Maggie Aderin-Pocock says.

3. Dyslexics have high levels of empathy.

It isn't just our knack of making complex ideas clearer that makes us strong communicators. We're also able to use our high levels of empathy and emotional intelligence to create messages that are compelling too.

Gareth Cook, a journalist who is made by dyslexia and writes for the *New York Times Magazine* and the *Boston Globe*, won the Pulitzer Prize in 2005 for "explaining, with clarity and humanity, the complex scientific and ethical dimensions of stem-cell research."

Dyslexics have a greater ability to sense, understand and respond to how others feel. This allows for a more authentic connection with

"Five Reasons Why Dyslexics Make Great Communicators"

people and can result in a deeper understanding of their stories and a greater skill in telling them. It's all part of our "Connecting" skills.

The Right Rev. Sarah Mullally, Bishop of London, recognizes the strengths her dyslexia brings: "I love listening and solving problems. I also have a high level of emotional intelligence. I will respond differently to situations than other people."

Empathy and emotional intelligence featured highly in Bishop Sarah's previous life, too. Before her ordination, she was the UK's Chief Nursing Officer. With these enhanced emotional strengths, it's no surprise that many dyslexics are drawn to careers like nursing, caring, social work and becoming champions of the socially disadvantaged. In fact, Dame Martina Milburn, Group Chief Executive of the Prince's Trust and Chair of the Social Mobility Commission, is also made by dyslexia.

4. Dyslexics are passionate and curious.

What really makes dyslexics amazing communicators is our passion and curiosity. We love learning new things. And the energy and passion we use to do it inspires others.

Jamie Oliver's infectious energy, and skill in communicating, has made even the most complex recipes simple and easy for most of us to have a go at in our own kitchens. In this way, he's able to pass on his passion and curiosity to millions of us around the world.

5. Dyslexics engage hearts and minds.

The combination of being able to make sense of the bigger picture, simplify complex ideas, use our emotional intelligence and inspire people with our passion and curiosity means we are great at engaging hearts and minds. We know how to entertain, inspire, motivate and influence people.

Dav Pilkey, the creator of Captain Underpants, says his dyslexia and other learning abilities "helped me to write stories that were not boring. It helped me to choose my words very, very carefully." His words (and pictures) have helped millions of children (dyslexic or not) love reading.

Appendix H
Helpful Links and Resources on Reading

Online Media

American Public Media's (APM) Reporting on Reading:
https://www.apmreports.org/reading
Audio versions of the APM Reports stories:

- *Educate* podcast
    - ◊ *https://www.apmreports.org/educate-podcast* (homepage)
    - ◊ *https://podcasts.apple.com/us/podcast/id81914987* (Apple Podcasts link)
- APM Reports Documentaries, podcast feed
    - ◊ *https://features.apmreports.org/podcasts/*

A discussion guide to accompany APM's "At a Loss for Words: What's Wrong with How Schools Teach Reading" is available from the Right to Read Project: *https://righttoreadproject.com/2019/08/27/discussion-guide-at-a-loss-for-words/*

Books

Stanislas Dehaene. *Reading in the Brain: The New Science of How We Read.* New York: Penguin, 2009.

- There are a number of videos on YouTube featuring Dehaene's work, including: *https://www.youtube.com/watch?v=wlYZBi_07vk*
- His lectures can be found on YouTube, as well: *https://www.youtube.com/watch?v=MSy685vNqYk https://www.youtube.com/watch?v=0esnsHI4opA*

David Kilpatrick. *Essentials of Assessing, Preventing, and Overcoming Reading Difficulties.* New York: Wiley, 2015.

Helpful Links and Resources on Reading

- This book includes a good explanation of orthographic mapping

Mark Seidenberg. *Language at the Speed of Sight.* New York: Basic Books, 2017.
- Seidenberg's website has many links and resources about the science of reading: *https://seidenbergreading.net/science-of-reading/*

Natalie Wexler. *The Knowledge Gap: The Hidden Cause of America's Broken Education System—and How to Fix It.* New York: Avery, 2019.
- Wexler writes a column for *Forbes* and frequently covers reading instruction: *https://www.forbes.com/sites/nataliewexler/#448ca89f4e29*

Articles and Other Resources

Anne Castles and Jennifer Buckingham. "Why Do Some Children Learn to Read Without Explicit Teaching?" *https://www.nomanis.com.au/post/why-do-some-children-learn-to-read-without-explicit-teaching*

Anne Castles, Kathy Rastle, and Kate Nation. "Ending the Reading Wars: Reading Acquisition from Novice to Expert." *Psychological Science in the Public Interest* 19, no. 1: 5–51. *https://www.psychologicalscience.org/publications/ending-the-reading-wars-reading-acquisition-from-novice-to-expert.html*
- This is a freely available, thorough overview of decades of scientific research on reading, full of citations.

Center for Early Reading. "Learning to Read: A Primer."
- Part 1: *http://go.info.amplify.com/hubfs/CFER/Primer/PrimerPt1_LearningToRead.pdf*
- Part 2: *https://go.info.amplify.com/hubfs/Primer%20II/Primer2_2018_Final.pdf*

Anne Cunningham and Keith Stanovich. "What Reading Does for the Mind." *Journal of Direct Instruction* 1, no. 2 (summer 2001): 137–149. *https://mccleskeyms.typepad.com/files/what-reading-does-for-the-mind.pdf*

Linda Farrell, Marcia Davidson, Michael Hunter, and Tina Osenga. "The Simple View of Reading." Center for Development and Learning (website). *https://www.cdl.org/the-simple-view-of-reading/*

Appendix H

Margaret Goldberg. "Teachers Won't Embrace Research Until It Embraces Them." *Right to Read Project* (blog). https://righttoreadproject.com/2019/07/19/teachers-wont-embrace-research-until-it-embraces-them/

Louisa Moats. "Teaching Reading Is Rocket Science: What Expert Teachers of Reading Should Know and Be Able to Do." https://www.aft.org/ae/summer2020/moats
- This is an updated version of a piece originally published in 1999.

Kate Nation and Jennifer Buckingham. "Learning to Read and Explicit Teaching." *Teacher* (website). https://www.teachermagazine.com.au/articles/learning-to-read-and-explicit-teaching

Laura Stewart. "The Science of Reading: Evidence for a New Era of Reading Instruction." White paper. Columbus, OH: Zaner-Bloser, 2020. https://iferi.org/wp-content/uploads/2020/03/Science-of-Reading-White-Paper-Stewart.pdf

Rebecca Treiman. "What Research Tells Us About Reading Instruction." *Psychological Science in the Public Interest* 19, no. 1 (2018): 1–4. https://journals.sagepub.com/doi/pdf/10.1177/1529100618772272

Sebastian Wren. "Ten Myths about Learning to Read." *Reading Rockets.* https://www.readingrockets.org/article/ten-myths-about-learning-read

Chapter Notes

Introduction

1. The 2004 Response to Intervention (RTI) process was introduced in the 2004 reauthorization of the Individuals with Disabilities Act (IDEA). Lauren Bates, Nicole Breslow, and Naomi Hupert, "Five States' Efforts to Improve Adolescent Literacy," Issues & Answers Report, REL 2009-No.067, 2009, https://ies.ed.gov/ncee/edlabs/regions/northeast/pdf/REL_2009067.pdf.

2. Dr. Sally Shaywitz, https://medicine.yale.edu/profile/sally_shaywitz.

3. Peter W. D. Wright, Esq., is an attorney with a degree in psychology and represents children with special education needs. See more on his Special Education Law and Advocacy Bootcamp conference training at www.wrightslaw.com.

4. Specific learning disabilities, as defined by the Individuals with Disabilities Education Act (IDEA) in 1975, include thirteen learning disabilities. https://sites.ed.gov/idea/about-idea/.

5. Individuals with Disabilities Education Act (IDEA), see Sec. 300.111, Child Find Act, https://sites.ed.gov/idea/regs/b/b/300.111.

6. Orton-Gillingham was pioneered in the 1930s and provided the foundation for student instruction and teacher training to focus attention on reading failure. https://www.ortonacademy.org/resources/what-is-the-orton-gillingham-approach/.

7. Rawson Sanders, Multisensory School, https://www.rawsonsaunders.org/about.

8. Linda Borg, on using the "D" word, in "Dyslexia at School: Advocates Push for Bill to Mandate Screen and Intervention," *Providence Journal*, May 31, 2016, https://www.providencejournal.com/article/20160531/NEWS/160539859.

9. Emily Hanford is a senior producer and education correspondent for APM Reports. In 2017, she won the Excellence in Media Reporting on Education Research Award. https://www.apmreports.org/emily-hanford.

10. The Reading Wars, a debate about the "best way" to teach reading, has been raging for decades. There are opposing factions of experts, policy makers, and politicians who champion "phonics," on the one side, or "whole language," on the other. "Beyond the Reading Wars: Embracing the Science of Learning," *Lexia*, https://www.lexialearning.com/blog/beyond-reading-wars-embracing-science-learning.

Chapter 1

1. "Definition of Dyslexia," adopted by the International Dyslexia Association Board of Directors, November 12, 2002, https://dyslexiaida.org/definition-of-dyslexia/.

2. Gavin R. Price and Daniel Ansari, "Dyscalculia: Characteristics, Causes, and Treatments," *Numeracy* 6, no. 1 (2013), http://scholarcommons.usf.edu/numeracy/vol6/iss1/art2.

3. Sheryl M. Handler, Walter M. Fierson, et al., "Learning Disabilities, Dyslexia, and Vision," *Pediatrics* 127, no. 3 (March 2011): e818–e856, https://pediatrics.aappublications.org/content/127/3/e818.short.

Notes—Chapter 1

4. IEE, http://cflparents.org/Infor mation/Resources/PublicSchool/Zirkel IEEArticle-April2009.pdf.

5. The Individuals with Disabilities Education Act, https://sites.ed.gov/idea/about-idea/.

6. Nadine Gaab, PhD, https://www.gaablab.com/nadine-gaab.

7. Nadine Gaab, PhD, "The Typical and Atypical Reading Brain: How a Neurobiological Framework of Reading Development Can Inform Educational Practices and Policy," http://www.decodingdyslexiama.org/uploads/1/8/5/1/18517104/dr._nadine_gaab_presen tation.pdf.

8. Anne Puolakanaho, et al., "Very Early Phonological and Language Skills: Estimating Individual Risk of Reading Disability," *The Journal of Child Psychology and Psychiatry* 48, no. 9 (September 2007): 923–931, https://onlinelibrary.wiley.com/doi/full/10.1111/j.1469-7610.2007.01763.x.

9. Todd L. Richards and Virginia W. Berninger, "Abnormal fMRI Connectivity in Children with Dyslexia during a Phoneme Task: Before But Not After Treatment," *Journal of Neurolinguistics* 21, no. 4 (July 2008): 294–304, https://dx.doi.org/10.1016%2Fj.jneuroling.2007.07.002.

10. P. H. T. Leppänen, et al., "Cortical Responses of Infants with and without a Genetic Risk for Dyslexia: II. Group Effects," *Cortex* 46 (2010): 1362–1376; Heikki Lyytinen, Jane Erskine, Jarmo Hämäläinen, Minna Torppa, and Miia Ronimus, "Dyslexia—Early Identification and Prevention: Highlights from the Jyväskylä Longitudinal Study of Dyslexia," *Current Developmental Disorders Reports* 2, no. 4 (2015): 330–338, https://www.ncbi.nlm.nih.gov/pmc/articles/PMC4624816/.

11. Lyytinen, Erskine, Hämäläinen, Torppa, and Ronimus, "Dyslexia—Early Identification and Prevention."

12. Free Appropriate Public Education for Students with Disabilities: Requirements Under Section 504 of the Rehabilitation Act of 1973, https://www2.ed.gov/about/offices/list/ocr/docs/edlite-FAPE504.html.

13. "Timeline of Learning Disabilities," *LD Online*, http://www.ldonline.org/article/11244/.

14. Shirley Carlson, "A Two-Hundred Year History of Learning Disabilities," November 17, 2005, https://files.eric.ed.gov/fulltext/ED490746.pdf, citing D. P. Hallahan and C. D. Mercer, "Learning Disabilities, Historical Perceptions. Executive Summary," 2001.

15. "History of Dyslexia Research," Wikipedia, https://en.wikipedia.org/wiki/History_of_dyslexia_research.

16. Steven A. Stahl and Patricia D. Miller, "Whole Language and Language Experience Approaches for Beginning Reading: A Quantitative Research Synthesis," *Review of Educational Research* 59, no. 1 (1989): 87–116, https://journals.sagepub.com/doi/10.3102/00346543059001087.

17. Bette S. Bergeron, "What Does the Term Whole Language Mean? Constructing a Definition from the Literature," *Journal of Reading Behavior* XXII, no. 4 (1990), https://journals.sagepub.com/doi/pdf/10.1080/10862969009547716.

18. G. Reid Lyon, "Why Reading Is Not a Natural Process," https://www.reidlyon.com/edpolicy/4-WHY-READING-IS-NOT-A-NATURAL-PROCESS.pdf.

19. Erica L. Green and Dana Goldstein, "Reading Scores on National Exam Decline in Half the States," *New York Times*, October 30, 2019, https://www.nytimes.com/2019/10/30/us/reading-scores-national-exam.html.

20. Jenifer Jasinski Schneider, "The Reading Wars," in *The Inside, Outside, and Upside Downs of Children's Literature: From Poets and Pop-ups to Princesses and Porridge* (Tampa, FL, University of South Florida: Teaching and Learning at Scholar Commons, 2016), 159–198, https://scholarcommons.usf.edu/cgi/viewcontent.cgi?referer=https://www.google.com/&httpsredir=1&article=1006&context=childrens_lit_textbook.

21. Emily Hanford, https://www.apmreports.org/emily-hanford.

22. Annie E. Casey Foundation, "Double Jeopardy: How Third Grade Reading Skills and Poverty Influence High

Notes—Chapter 2

School Graduation," Report, January 1, 2012, https://www.aecf.org/resources/double-jeopardy/.

23. "Essential Qualities of a Good Journalist," Reva University, https://reva.edu.in/blog/essential-qualities-of-a-good-journalist/.

Chapter 2

1. For more on media effects theory, see Jennings Bryant and Mary Beth Oliver, eds., *Media Effects: Advances in Theory and Research*, 3rd ed. (London: Routledge, 2008).

2. This term and concept is often used to describe the nonrepresentation, which has psychological ramifications for people by gender, race, ethnicity, or, we would argue, disability. The earliest studies were done by the sociologist Gaye Tuchman, who described the phenomenon as "a process by which the mass media omit, trivialize, or condemn certain groups that are not socially valued." Hugh Klein and Kenneth S. Shiffman, "Underrepresentation and Symbolic Annihilation of Social Disenfranchised Groups ('Out Groups') in Animated Cartoons," *Howard Journal of Communications* 10, no. 1 (2009): 55–72, https://www.ncbi.nlm.nih.gov/pmc/articles/PMC6124697/.

3. "Making Contact—Why Media Is Important," *Our Community*, https://www.ourcommunity.com.au/marketing/marketing_article.jsp?articleId=1593.

4. Lexi Walters Wright, "10 Movie and TV Characters with Dyslexia," *Understood*, https://www.understood.org/en/learning-thinking-differences/child-learning-disabilities/dyslexia/10-movie-and-tv-characters-with-dyslexia. All references, unless otherwise noted, are taken from this source.

5. Sue Corsall, "The Portrayal of Learning Disabilities in the Media," *The Portrayal of Disabilities in the Media* (blog), June 3, 2013, https://suecorsall.wordpress.com/2013/06/03/the-portrayal-of-learning-disabilities-in-the-media/.

6. Quoted from Kathy Crocket, "Jay Leno, Comedian and Television Personality," Yale Center for Dyslexia and Creativity, https://dyslexia.yale.edu/story/jay-leno/.

7. Associated Press, "Dyslexia More Common in Boys, Study Finds," *NBC News*, April 27, 2004, https://www.nbcnews.com/health/health-news/dyslexia-more-common-boys-study-finds-flna1c9444793.

8. "L Is for dyslexia," *TV Tropes*, https://tvtropes.org/pmwiki/pmwiki.php/Main/LIsForDyslexia.

9. Emilie S. Peck, "Top Four Dyslexia Documentary Movies," *Reel Rundown*, March 8, 2018, https://reelrundown.com/movies/Top-Four-Dyslexia-Documentary-Movies.

10. Manpreet Singh, "Top 10 Inspirational Movies on Dyslexia, Number Dyslexia," *Number Dyslexia*, July 20, 2019, http://numberdyslexia.com/top-8-inspirational-movies-on-dyslexia/.

11. Stella Young, "We're Not Here for Your Inspiration," *Ramp Up* (blog), July 2, 2012, http://www.abc.net.au/rampup/articles/2012/07/02/3537035.htm.

12. See the full text, as well as the video of Young's speech here: https://www.ted.com/talks/stella_young_i_m_not_your_inspiration_thank_you_very_much/transcript.

13. David Williams, "Undefeated Wrestler Lets Opponent with Down Syndrome Win," *CNN*, January 28, 2016, https://www.cnn.com/2016/01/28/us/undefeated-wrestler-down-syndrome-irpt/.

14. "Very Special Homecoming King and Queen Crowned at Tri-West," YouTube, February 10, 2014, https://www.youtube.com/watch?v=PXQq2EU6-zs.

15. Eileen Daily, "'Inspiration Porn' Trending on Social Media Is Objectification of Disabled People," *The Journal.ie*, February 12, 2019, https://www.thejournal.ie/readme/opinion-stop-sharing-videos-of-disabled-people-attempting-to-walk-up-the-aisle-or-stand-for-their-first-dance-that-is-far-from-inspirational-4489295-Feb2019/.

16. Saidee Wynn, "Please Stop Spreading 'Inspiration Porn' about Disability," *The Mighty*, October 2, 2017, https://

Notes—Chapter 3

themighty.com/2017/10/please-stop-spreading-inspiration-porn-about-disability/.

17. K. Mead, "How the Media and Society Objectify Disabled People," *Paginated Thoughts* (blog), September 5, 2016, https://kpagination.wordpress.com/2016/09/05/how-media-and-society-objectify-disabled-people/.

18. Amy S. F. Lutz, "Bring on the 'Inspiration Porn,'" *Psychology Today*, October 19, 2016, https://www.psychologytoday.com/us/blog/inspectrum/201610/bring-the-inspiration-porn.

19. David M. Perry, "How 'Inspiration Porn' Reporting Objectifies People with Disabilities," *Medium*, February 25, 2016, https://medium.com/the-establishment/how-inspiration-porn-reporting-objectifies-people-with-disabilities-db30023e3d2b.

Chapter 3

1. Speech given by Fred Friendly at the Hamilton School at Wheeler, Providence, Rhode Island, April 7, 1995, quote from p. 1. Typescript retrieved from the archives of the Hamilton School at Wheeler. Also available in the Fred Friendly Collection in the archives of Columbia University.

2. Ralph Engelman, *Friendlyvision: Fred Friendly and the Rise and Fall of Television Journalism* (New York: Columbia University Press, 1995), 20. Much of the background on Fred Friendly's life, unless otherwise cited as first-person from interviews with the authors, derives from Engleman's biography, with the more important areas designated with page numbers.

3. Engelman, *Friendlyvision*, 16.
4. Engelman, *Friendlyvision*, 17.
5. Engelman, *Friendlyvision*, 11
6. Engelman, *Friendlyvision*, 23.

7. In his 1995 speech at the Hamilton School at Wheeler, on p. 2 of the typescript, Friendly referred to the poem and his aunt's involvement in the title of the *Footprints* programs, stating, "My aunt gave me a way to begin the program with lines from a famous poem by Henry Wadsworth Longfellow called, 'Psalm of Life.' The lines:
Lives of great men all remind us
We can make our lives sublime
And departing leave behind us
Footprints on the sands of time."

8. Hamilton School at Wheeler speech, p. 2 of typescript.

9. Hamilton School at Wheeler speech, p. 2 of typescript.

10. The history of Fred Friendly's military experiences are detailed in Engelman, *Friendlyvision*, Chapter 2, "My Rhodes Scholarship," 30–47, and is the principal source for this period in his life.

11. Engelman, *Friendlyvision*, 37.

12. Engelman, *Friendlyvision*, 36–39, contains Major Clark's praise of Fred Friendly's achievements while in the army's Office of Information and Education.

13. Hamilton School at Wheeler speech, p. 3 of typescript.

14. Engelman, *Friendlyvision*, 46.

15. In Engelman's biography, there's an account of how "at the end of the war, Friendly had declaimed to Major Clark the importance of recorders for the future of communications. Immediately after the war audio technology took a leap forward; the old wire-recording system was replaced by magnetic audio tape, which created new possibilities for the editing of audio." Engelman, *Friendlyvision*, 56.

16. The Friendly–Murrow collaborative partnership, beginning with radio and continuing in television, is detailed in several Murrow biographies, including A. M. Sperber, *Murrow: His Life and Times* (New York: Fordham University Press, 1986); Joseph E. Persico, *Edward R. Murrow: An American Original* (New York: McGraw-Hill, 1988); and Bob Edwards, *Edward R. Murrow and the Birth of Broadcast Journalism* (Hoboken, NJ: John Wiley & Sons, 2004).

17. Fred Friendly wrote, among his four published books, one book in particular that chronicled the *See It Now* broadcast involving Senator McCarthy, titled *Due to Circumstances Beyond Our Control* (New York: Vintage, 1968).

18. Personal interview with Ruth Mark Friendly, June 30, 2019. Future references

Notes—Chapter 4

to comments by Mrs. Friendly are taken from the transcript of this interview.

19. Hamilton School at Wheeler speech, p. 1 of typescript.

20. Personal interview with Lisa Friendly, July 12, 2019. Future references to comments by Ms. Friendly are taken from the transcript of this interview.

21. Details of Fred Friendly's later years at the Ford Foundation and Columbia University and founding PBS are summarized in Engelman, *Friendlyvision*, Chapter 20, "The Last Years," 329–345.

22. Hamilton School at Wheeler speech, p. 4 of typescript.

23. Hamilton School at Wheeler speech, p. 4 of typescript.

Chapter 4

1. Anderson Cooper did not agree to a personal interview for this book, so the material contained in this chapter is from secondary sources, including articles he has written, lectures he has given, or interviews done elsewhere in which he is quoted on the subject of dyslexia.

2. For a biography of Cooper, see "Anderson Cooper Biography," *Encyclopedia of World Biography*, https://www.notablebiographies.com/newsmakers2/2006-A-Ec/Cooper-Anderson.html, where much of his early family life is detailed, in addition to his career path to CNN.

3. From an address given at the National Center for Learning Disabilities Annual Luncheon, New York, November 22, 2010, https://www.youtube.com/watch?v=prNSvErKQug.

4. An overview of this topic is found in Shane Herman, "Why Dyslexics Have Low Self-Confidence," *Let's Get Booking*, September 3, 2018, https://www.letsgetbooking.com/why-dyslexics-have-low-self-confidence/.

5. Cooper once wrote about the relationship with his famous mother in *The Rainbow Comes and Goes: A Mother and Son on Life, Love, and Loss* (New York: Harper, 2016).

6. Eric Sumner, "The Remarkable True Story Behind Anderson Cooper's Explosive Career," *Direct Expose*, July 4, 2019, https://www.directexpose.com/true-story-anderson-cooper/2/.

7. Cooper's early reading choices, as well as those later in his life, are detailed in "Books that Made a Difference to Anderson Cooper," *O Magazine*, http://www.oprah.com/omagazine/anderson-coopers-books-that-made-a-difference, and "Anderson Cooper's Bookshelf," *O Magazine*, http://www.oprah.com/omagazine/Anderson-Coopers-Bookshelf/1.

8. Cooper was describing his attraction to Conrad's *Heart of Darkness*. "Anderson's Favorite Books," *All Things Anderson Cooper*, http://www.allthingsandersoncooper.com/2010/02/andersons-favorite-books.html.

9. "Anderson Cooper," *Biography*, January 4, 2018, https://www.biography.com/media-figure/anderson-cooper. This site also contains information about Cooper's coping with loss after his brother's untimely death. He also raises the same question in "Anderson Cooper," *Standing Tall with Dyslexia*, October 18, 2018, https://sites.psu.edu/mrjpassion/2018/10/18/6-anderson-cooper/.

10. Stephen Matthews, "Anderson Cooper Visits Colorado to Listen to Colorado Students," *La Junta Tribune-Democrat*, March 9, 2018, https://www.lajuntatribunedemocrat.com/news/20180309/anderson-cooper-visits?template=ampart.

11. Ellen Cranley, "The Incredible Life of Anderson Cooper: How the Son of an Heiress Became America's Favorite News Anchor," *Business Insider*, June 28, 2019.

12. Much of the information about Cooper's rise from Channel One to ABC and CNN is found on his Wikipedia page, https://en.wikipedia.org/wiki/Anderson_Cooper#Channel_One.

13. Anderson Cooper, *Dispatches from the Edge: A Memoir of War, Disasters, and Survival* (New York: Harper, 2006).

14. Learning Disabilities Association of Alberta, Facebook post, September 1, 2019, https://www.facebook.com/LearningDisabilitiesNL/posts/2520458308013762.

15. Jonathan Capehart, "Anderson Cooper Out in the Open," *Washington Post*, July 3, 2012, https://www.washingtonpost.com/blogs/post-partisan/post/anderson-cooper-out-in-the-open/2012/07/03/gJQAwv5eKW_blog.html.

Chapter 5

1. From personal interview with the authors, October 11, 2019. Unless otherwise noted, quotations are taken from this interview.
2. Neal Conan, "Byron Pitts Found Faith to 'Step Out on Nothing,'" *Talk of the Nation*, National Public Radio, November 16, 2009, https://www.npr.org/transcripts/120463986.
3. Al Tomkpins, "CBS' Byron Pitts Details Childhood Illiteracy in New Memoir," *Poynter*, September 14, 2009, https://www.poynter.org/reporting-editing/2009/cbs-byron-pitts-details-childhood-illiteracy-in-new-memoir/.
4. Quoted from "The Stuttering Foundation" website, https://www.stutteringhelp.org/famous-people/byron-pitts-0. This is the source for much of the background on stuttering, but Pitts himself discusses his stuttering problems in Byron Pitts, *Step Out on Nothing: How Faith and Family Helped Me Conquer Life's Challenges* (New York: St. Martin's Press, 2009).
5. Tompkins, "CBS' Byron Pitts Details Childhood Illiteracy in New Memoir."
6. From personal correspondence, June 12, 2020.
7. "Byron Pitts Talks Family, Faith, Dreams in MLK Commemoration Speech," Student Leadership and Engagement, NC State University, October 31, 2015, https://studentinvolvement.dasa.ncsu.edu/byron-pitts-mlk-commemoration-spech/.
8. Tompkins, "CBS' Byron Pitts Details Childhood Illiteracy in New Memoir."
9. Bonnie Duncan, "Pitts Discusses Journalism Experience," *The Hoya*, December 4, 2009, https://thehoya.com/pitts-discusses-journalism-experience/.

Chapter 6

1. She writes about her home country in an article titled "A Correspondent's Take on Johannesburg," *CNN*, April 19, 2010, https://www.cnn.com/2010/TRAVEL/04/09/curnow.johannesburg.travel/index.html.
2. From her official biography, https://www.cnn.com/CNN/anchors_reporters/curnow.robyn.html.
3. Robyn Curnow, "The Upside to Dyslexia, Even as a Journalist," *CNN*, June 6, 2019, https://www.cnn.com/2019/06/06/health/dyslexia-benefit-curnow/index.html.
4. She writes about this experience in detail in "'I Realized I Was Dyslexic When My Daughter Was Diagnosed,'" *Indian Express*, October 22, 2019, https://indianexpress.com/article/parenting/blog/i-realised-i-was-dyslexic-when-my-daughter-was-diagnosed-6079890/.
5. From personal interviews with the authors in fall 2019 and March 2020. Much of the material in this chapter derives from those interviews, but some is also contained in articles written by Robyn Curnow in which she conveys the same material. Where the secondary reference is important, it is cited. Otherwise, its source is the aforementioned interviews.
6. Robyn Curnow, "A Candidate for Governor of Maryland Stutters. So Does My Young Daughter," September 9, 2018, *Washington Post*, washingtonpost.com/outlook/2018/09/10/candidate-governor-maryland-stutters-so-does-my-young-daughter/.
7. Much of this section is attributable to personal interviews, as well as Robyn Curnow's video interview, #madebydyslexia, Facebook post, October 7, 2019, https://www.facebook.com/madebydyslexia/videos/399881547348937/?v=399881547348937.
8. Sentiments expressed in personal interviews, "The Upside to Dyslexia," as well as in the NPR interview, "CNN's Robyn Curnow Says Dyslexia Can Be an Asset," November 1, 2019, https://www.gpbnews.org/post/cnns-robyn-curnow-says-dyslexia-can-be-asset.

9. From Curnow, "The Upside to Dyslexia."
10. Robyn Curnow, "The World Is Waking Up to the Power of Dyslexia," *Africa Business Communities*, November 10, 2019, https://africabusinesscommunities.com/features/column-robyn-curnow-the-world-is-waking-up-to-the-power-of-dyslexia/.
11. Curnow, "The Upside to Dyslexia."

Chapter 7

1. Orton-Gillingham, an approach to reading developed in the 1930s, as described on Wikipedia, https://en.wikipedia.org/wiki/Orton-Gillingham.
2. Walcott School, Chicago, Illinois, https://wolcottschool.org/.
3. Hyde Park Day School, Chicago, Illinois, http://hydeparkday.org/.
4. "Ida B. Wells," *Biography*, https://www.biography.com/activist/ida-b-wells.
5. "Nellie Bly," *Biography*, https://www.biography.com/activist/nellie-bly.
6. "Five Reasons Why a Google Doodle Tribute to Nellie Bly Is Justified," *Biharprabha*. May 5, 2015, https://news.biharprabha.com/2015/05/five-reasons-why-a-google-doodle-tribute-to-nellie-bly-is-justified/.
7. *American Experience*, PBS.
8. Debra Bradley Ruder, "Street Doctor," *Harvard University Magazine*, January–February 2016, https://harvardmagazine.com/2016/01/street-doctor.
9. Rhodes Project website, http://rhodesproject.com/.

Chapter 8

1. From Jill Wellington, LinkedIn, https://www.linkedin.com/in/jill-wellington-75707755.
2. From personal interview with Jill Wellington, done by authors, October 30, 2019. All subsequent quotations are from this interview, unless otherwise noted.
3. Jill Wellington, "How I Overcame Dyslexia to Become a Journalist," *Holistic Shop*, 2004, https://www.holisticshop.co.uk/articles/life-mission-heart. This section and others in the chapter that aren't specifically from the authors' interviews are attributable to this source, unless otherwise noted.
4. Helen Robinson, "Getting to Know You: Behind the Lens with Jill Wellington," *Topaz Labs Behind the Lens* (blog), February 12, 2017, http://blog.topazlabs.com/getting-to-know-jill-wellington/.
5. From Jill Wellington, LinkedIn, https://www.linkedin.com/in/jill-wellington-75707755.

Chapter 9

1. From personal interview with the authors. Quotations are from this source, unless otherwise noted.
2. He also discusses his childhood experiences and frustrations with dyslexia in other sources, including an interview with the Yale Center for Dyslexia and Creativity: Jane Wallace, "Success Stories: Richard Engel, Chief Foreign Correspondent for NBC News," https://dyslexia.yale.edu/story/richard-engel/.
3. For more on Richard Engel's views on becoming successful with dyslexia, see Rachel Ehmke, "Richard Engel on Finding Success with Dyslexia," Child Mind Institute, https://childmind.org/article/richard-engel-on-finding-success-with-dyslexia/.
4. Additional background on Richard Engel's childhood dyslexia and his coping mechanisms can be found in "High Achieving Dyslexics: Richard Engel, Journalist," *I Speak in Dreams*, November 29, 2006, https://lizditz.typepad.com/i_speak_of_dreams/2006/11/high_achieving_.html.
5. Engel has been profiled in a series focusing on ongoing successful individuals with dyslexia in "Dyslexia: The Gift," Davis Dyslexia Association International, https://www.dyslexia.com/famous/richard-engel/.
6. Engel has detailed the challenges his young son faces in Anika Reed, "NBC Correspondent Richard Engel Gets Emotional after Son with Rett Syndrome Says 'Dada,'" *USA Today*, March 15, 2019, https://www.usatoday.com/story/life/allthemoms/2019/03/15/nbc-richard-

Notes—Chapters 10 and 11

engel-son-rett-syndrome-says-dada-writes-emotional-essay/3175071002/.

Chapter 10

1. From an interview with the authors, June 20, 2020. All citations are from this source, unless otherwise noted.

2. APM Reports, "Stuck at Square One," 2016, https://www.apmreports.org/files/StuckAtSquareOne.pdf.

3. The purpose of this test, according to the company's website, is "to evaluate the mathematics, reading and writing skills of test-takers. Some individuals may also take the Accuplacer tests during high school to determine if they are ready to pursue postsecondary studies or to identify areas where they need to improve to be ready for college." Sandra Lindenmuth, "What Is the Accuplacer Test?," *Study.com*, https://study.com/academy/popular/what-is-the-accuplacer-test.html#:~:text=The%20purpose%20of%20the%20Accuplacer,to%20be%20ready%20for%20college.

4. "Science of Reading: Conversation with Emily Hanford," *Amplify Education* (podcast), November 13, 2019, http://www.buzzsprout.com/612361/1963279-a-conversation-with-emily-hanford.

5. Emily Hanford, "Hard to Read: How American Schools Fail Kids with Dyslexia," *APM Reports*, September 11, 2017, https://www.apmreports.org/story/2017/09/11/hard-to-read.

6. Dr. Jack M. Fletcher, "Understanding Dyslexia and Its Implications for Identification and Treatment," Center for Learning & Disabilities, University of Houston, https://21tb7c2uredpvu4mah6gyjmt-wpengine.netdna-ssl.com/assets/summit2017/JackFletcher.pdf.

7. Sara Briggs, "The Matthew Effect: What Is It and How Can You Avoid It in Your Classroom?" *informED*, July 1, 2013, https://www.opencolleges.edu.au/informed/features/the-matthew-effect-what-is-it-and-how-can-you-avoid-it-in-your-classroom/.

8. Emily Hanford, "American Schools Are Failing Students with Dyslexia: What Can We Do About It?," Voyager Sopris Learning, *EdView 360* (podcast), October 22, 2019, https://www.voyagersopris.com/podcast/emily-hanford.

9. Phonics is defined as "a method of teaching people to read by correlating sounds with letters or groups of letters in an alphabetic writing system." *Your Dictionary*, https://www.yourdictionary.com/phonics.

10. Lucy Calkins, Teachers College Reading and Writing Project, Wikipedia, https://en.wikipedia.org/wiki/Teachers_College_Reading_and_Writing_Project.

11. See Valerie Strauss, "A Case for Why Both Sides in the Reading Wars Are Wrong—And a Proposed Solution," *Washington Post*, March 27, 2019, https://www.washingtonpost.com/education/2019/03/27/case-why-both-sides-reading-wars-debate-are-wrong-proposed-solution/. Also, Jill Barshay, "Four Things You Need to Know About the New Reading Wars," *The Hechinger Report*, March 30, 2020, https://hechingerreport.org/four-things-you-need-to-know-about-the-new-reading-wars/. An earlier report on the "Reading Wars" is found in Nicholas Leman, "The Reading Wars: An Old Disagreement Over How to Teach Children to Read—Whole Language versus Phonics," *The Atlantic*, November 1997, https://www.theatlantic.com/magazine/archive/1997/11/the-reading-wars/376990/.

12. Tim Odegard, PhD, CALP, Middle Tennessee State University, Center for Dyslexia, Tennessee Center for the Study and Treatment of Dyslexia, https://www.mtsu.edu/dyslexia/staff.php.

Chapter 11

1. Yale Center for Dyslexia and Creativity, https://dyslexia.yale.edu/.

2. Simulation online, https://geon.github.io/programming/2016/03/03/dsxyliea.

3. *Independent* online dyslexia coverage, https://www.independent.co.uk/topic/dyslexia.

4. Sarah, Duchess of York Charity, https://thedukeofyork.org/about-the-duke/princess-beatrice/.

Notes—Chapter 11

5. Shannon Heffernan, "6 Tips for Covering People with Disabilities," Poynter, July 24, 2015, https://www.poynter.org/reporting-editing/2015/6-tips-for-covering-people-with-disabilities/.

6. National Center on Disability and Journalism, "Disability Language Style Guide," https://ncdj.org/style-guide/.

7. CBS News, "Cracking the Code of Dyslexia," *CBS News*, https://www.cbsnews.com/news/cracking-the-code-of-dyslexia/.

8. Parvati Shallow, "The Font that Could Help Dyslexics Read Better," *CBS News*, https://www.cbsnews.com/news/the-font-that-helps-dyslexics-read-better/.

9. Understood, "Do Dyslexia Fonts Help?" *Understood*, https://www.understood.org/en/learning-thinking-differences/child-learning-disabilities/dyslexia/dyslexia-friendly-font.

10. For more, see Keri Wilmot, "Omoguru," *Common Sense Media*, https://www.commonsensemedia.org/app-reviews/omoguru.

11. From a personal interview with Sarah Gross, June 15, 2020.

12. Vanessa Ho, "'I Have Dyslexia': A Chief Engineer Spoke Up to Help Others with Learning Disabilities," Microsoft, September 30, 2019, https://news.microsoft.com/features/i-have-dyslexia-chief-engineer-spoke-up-help-others-learning-disabilities/.

13. "Dyslexia in the News," Yale Center for Dyslexia and Creativity, http://dyslexia.yale.edu/category/dyslexia-in-the-news/.

14. "Press Kit," Yale Center for Dyslexia and Creativity, http://dyslexia.yale.edu/news-press/press-kit/.

15. "Covering Disability Issues," Society of Professional Journalists, https://www.spj.org/dtb5.asp.

16. NBC News, "'Spring Awakening' Offers Opportunity for Deaf Actors to Sign and Sing," *NBC News*, January 4, 2016, https://www.nbcnews.com/nightly-news/video/-spring-awakening—offers-opportunity-for-deaf-actors-to-sign-and-sing-595710019951.

17. Steve Hartman, "How a Couple with Down Syndrome Proved Critics Wrong," August 16, 2019, https://www.cbsnews.com/video/how-a-couple-with-down-syndrome-proved-critics-wrong/.

Select Bibliography

Borg, Linda. "Dyslexia at School: Advocates Push for Bill to Mandate Screening and Intervention." *Providence Journal*, May 31, 2016.
Compton, Donald L., et al. "Selecting At-Risk First-Grade Readers for Early Intervention: Eliminating False Positives and Exploring the Promise of a Two-Stage Gated Screening Process." *Journal of Educational Psychology* 102, no. 2 (2010): 327–340.
Cooper, Anderson. *Dispatches from the Edge: A Memoir of Wars, Disaster, and Survival.* New York: Harper, 2007.
_____. *The Rainbow Comes and Goes: A Mother and Son On Life, Love, and Loss.* New York: Harper, 2016.
Curnow, Robyn. "The Upside to Dyslexia, Even as a Journalist." *CNN*, June 6, 2019. https://www.cnn.com/2019/06/06/health/dyslexia-benefit-curnow/index.html.
_____. "The World Is Waking Up to the Power of Dyslexia." *CEO Africa*, October 13, 2019. https://www.ceoafrica.co.ke/the-world-is-waking-up-to-the-power-of-dyslexia/.
Edwards, Bob. *Edward R. Murrow and the Birth of Broadcast Journalism.* Hoboken, NJ: John Wiley and Sons, 2004.
Eide, Brock L., and Fernette F. Eide. *The Dyslexic Advantage: Unlocking the Hidden Potential of the Dyslexic Brain.* New York: Penguin Random House, 2012.
Emanuel, Gabrielle. "Unlocking Dyslexia." *NPR*, December 10, 2016. https://www.npr.org/sections/ed/2016/12/10/502601738/unlocking-dyslexia-personal-stories-of-frustration-and-success.
Engel, Richard. *And Then All Hell Broke Loose: Two Decades in the Middle East.* New York: Simon & Schuster, 2016.
_____. *A Fist in the Hornet's Nest: On the Ground in Baghdad, Before, During, and After the War.* New York: Hachette, 2005.
_____. *War Journal: My Five Years in Iraq.* New York: Simon & Schuster, 2008.
Engleman, Ralph. *Friendly Vision: Fred Friendly and the Rise and Fall of Television Journalism.* New York: Columbia University Press, 2011.
Fletcher, Jack M., G. Reid Lyon, Lynn S. Fuchs, and Marcia A. Barnes. *Learning Disabilities: From Identification to Intervention.* 2d ed. New York: Guilford, 2018.
Friendly, Fred. *Due to Circumstances Beyond Our Control....* New York: Vintage Books, 1968.
_____. *The Good Guys, the Bad Guys, and the First Amendment: Free Speech vs. Fairness in Broadcasting.* New York: Random House, 1976.
Fuchs, Douglas, et al. "Smart RTI: A Next-Generation Approach to Multilevel Prevention." *Exceptional Children* 78, no. 3 (2012): 263–279.
Hanford, Emily. "At a Loss for Words How a Flawed Idea Is Teaching Millions of Kids

Select Bibliography

to Be Poor Readers." *APM Reports*, August 22, 2019. https://www.apmreports.org/episode/2019/08/22/whats-wrong-how-schools-teach-reading.

———. "Hard to Read: How American Schools Fail Kids with Dyslexia." *APM Reports*, September 11, 2017. https://www.apmreports.org/episode/2017/09/11/hard-to-read.

———. "Hard Words: Why Aren't Kids Being Taught to Read?" *APM Reports*, September 10, 2018. https://www.apmreports.org/episode/2018/09/10/hard-words-why-american-kids-arent-being-taught-to-read.

Hayter, David. "What Does Dyslexia Mean to Me?" *Read and Spell* (blog), 2017. https://www.readandspell.com/us/what-does-dyslexia-mean.

Hayward, Will. "Journalist Who Overcame Dyslexia to Become Reporter Named Best in Wales." *Medium Corporation*, March 24, 2019.

Joshi, R. Malt Maletesha, Emily S. Binks-Cantrell, Lori Graham, Emily Ocker-Dean, Dennie L. Smith, and Regina Gooden. "Do Textbooks Used in University Reading Education Courses Conform to the Instructional Recommendations of the National Reading Panel?" *Journal of Learning Disabilities* 42, no. 5 (2009): 458–463.

Norton, Elizabeth S., and Maryanne Wolf. "Rapid Automatized Naming (RAN) and Reading Fluency: Implications for Understanding and Treatment of Reading Disabilities." *Annual Review of Psychology* 63, no. 1 (2012): 427–452.

Pitts, Byron. *Be the One: Six True Stories of Teens Overcoming Hardship with Hope.* New York: Simon & Schuster, 2017.

———. *Step Out on Nothing: How Faith and Family Helped Me Conquer Life's Challenges.* New York: St. Martin's Press, 2010.

Shaywitz, Sally. *Overcoming Dyslexia: A New and Complete Science-Based Program for Reading Problems at Any Level.* New York: Alfred A. Knopf, 2004.

Silvia, Tony. "Fred Friendly in Providence." *RI Jewish Historical Association Notes* 18, no. 1 (2019): 24–35.

Ugochukwu, Paula. "What It's Like to Be Diagnosed with Dyslexia as an Adult." *Metro*, February 23, 2019. https://metro.co.uk/2019/02/23/what-its-like-to-be-diagnosed-with-a-learning-disability-as-an-adult-8636996/.

Van Stone, Meagan. "I'm a Journalism Major and I'm Dyslexic." *Odyssey*, July 11, 2016. https://www.theodysseyonline.com/journalism-major-and-dyslexic.

Wellington, Jill. "How I Overcame Dyslexia to Become a Journalist." *Holistic Shop*. 2004. https://www.holisticshop.co.uk/articles/life-mission-heart.

Wright, Peter W. D., and Pamela Darr Wright. *From Emotions to Advocacy: The Special Education Survival Guide.* 2d ed. Hartfield, VA: Harbor House Law, 2006.

Index

ABC News (network) 62, 64
ADHD (Attention Deficit Disorder) 21, 116
Alfonsi, Sharyn 74
American Public Media 25, 129
Ann E. Casey Foundation 26
Anya's Bell (1999) 36
APM Reports 25, 126–127, 170
Associated Press 73, 145

Be the One: Six True Stories of Teens Overcoming Hardship with Hope 70
Beverly Hills 90210 (1990–2000) 32
Big Picture (concept) 1, 35, 45, 91
The Big Picture: Rethinking Dyslexia (2012) 35
Bly, Nellie 99, 108
Boston Children's Hospital 19
Branson, Sir Richard 17, 74–75, 93, 142, 166, 164, 167–168
broadcast journalism 71, 73, 111–112

CBS (network) 42, 52, 55, 64, 72, 74, 148–149
CIA (Central Intelligence Agency) 61
CNN (network) 57, 62–63, 79–80, 92, 147
Columbia University Graduate School of Journalism 42–43, 55
co-morbid data 18, 18, 21
Conrad, Joseph 59
Cooper, Wyatt Emory 59
Corsall, Susan 30–31
The Cosby Show (1989) 31

Dalton School 60
Daly, Ellen 30–40
A Death in the Family 60
Decca Records 52
Decoding Dyslexia (organization) 3, 13, 21

Diagnostic and Statistical Manual of Mental Disorders 18
Disabilities Education Act 19
disability 17, 125–126, 150
Dispatches from the Edge: A Memoir of War, Disasters, and Survival 62
Don't Call Me Stupid (2010) 35
Dyscalculia 18
dyslexia 17–18, 19, 21–24, 27
Dyslexia Awareness Month 5

early risk identification 18
Eden, Guinevere 101
educational psychology 19
Embracing Dyslexia (2013) 35
Emmy award 1, 72–73
evidence-based remediation 21
evidence-based systematic learning 13

Fishburne, Laurence 77
Footprints on the Sands of Time (radio series) 48–49, 52
Forhan, Margaret 44
Francis, Dr. Don 56
Free and Appropriate Public Education (FAPE) 21
Friendly, Lisa 54–55
Friendly, Ruth 4, 43, 47, 50, 52–53, 55–56
functionally illiterate 64–66, 134

Gabb, Dr. Nadine 19–20
Gall, Franz Joseph 24
General Hospital (1990) 31
The George Lopez Show (2002–2007) 32
Ginsberg, Allen 29
Greenberg, Hank 45
Grey's Anatomy (2005) 31–32
Gross, Sarah 147
Gude, J.G. (nicknamed Jap) 52

Index

Hamilton School at Wheeler 14, 43, 45, 56
Hanford, Emily 25, 126
Harris, Jill 127–128
Hartman, Steve 149
Harvard Medical School 19
HBO 34–35
Hear It Now 42, 49, 52–53
Heart of Darkness 59
Heathcote School 53
heredity 72
Hinshelwood, James 22
Hope Street High School 45

Independent Education Evaluation (IEE) 19
Individuals with Disabilities Education Act (IDEA) 19, 158, 160
inspiration porn 37
International Dyslexia Association 17

Jennison, James 48

Kapp, Jack 52
KDKA 48
Keller, Helen 60
kindergarten study (of dyslexics) 20, 24–5
Koester, Nicole 145–146

Leno, Jay 33, 166
Lewes, Ulle 70
Like Stars on Earth (2007) 34
Linares, Maya 148
Love, Mary (1985) 36
Lowe, Mowry 49
Lutz, Amy 40

Made By Dyslexia (organization) 1, 2, 91, 93
Mandela, Nelson 79, 89
Marconi, Guglielmo 48
McCarthy, Sen. Joseph 53
McGinley, John C. 69
McLuhan, Marshall 29
Mead, Kit 40
media coverage of dyslexics 9
mentally retarded 4, 64, 67
Miles, Haven 9
A Mind of Her Own (2006) 37
Mr. Providence 50
Mitra, Melanie 97–98
Murrow, Edward R. 4, 42, 52–53, 55, 57
My So-Called Life (1994) 32

National Association of Black Journalists 73
National Center for Family Literacy 66, 77
National Center for Learning Disabilities 23, 57–58
National Center on Disability and Journalism (NCDJ) 144–146
National Institute of Mental Health 23
National Institutes of Child Health and Human Development 17
NBC Nightly News 114, 123, 125, 149
neurology testing 19
New York Times 44, 68, 117, 139, 147, 168
news coverage of dyslexia 38–9, 41
Nichols College 47
Nightline 64–65, 74
North Carolina State University 73, 75
NPR (National Public Radio) 65, 95, 101–102, 106, 148, 151, 155, 158

Odegard, Tim 138
Ohio Wesleyan University 68–71
Omoguru (app) 147
Overcoming Dyslexia 11

PBS 42, 55
Peck, E.S. 34–36
Perry, David 41, 144
phonetic decoding 27
phonics 27, 135
Pilar 75
Pitts, Clarice 64, 67, 75–76
Poitier, Sydney 68
The Power of Positive Thinking 66
Poynter Institute for Media Studies 143
The Princess and the Cabbie (1981) 36
Providence Children's Center 4
Providence Journal 14
Providence Public Library 46

qualities of good journalism 25
Quinnipiac University 50

Remedial Reading Program 66
Rhode Island School for the Deaf 45
Rhodes Project 101
Riverdale Country School 115
Roberts, Cokie 73

Schneck School 81–83
The Secret (1992) 36
See It Now 42, 52–53
Shake It Up (2010–2013) 33

Index

60 Minutes 57, 62, 64, 73–74
Society of Professional Journalists (SPJ) 149–150
South African Broadcasting Company 79, 89–90
Step Out on Nothing: How Faith and Family Helped Me Conquer Life's Challenges 70
Streets of the City 49
stuttering 64–69, 71–72, 77
symbolic annihilation 30

teacher training, universities 20–21
Tonight Show/Jay Leno (1992–2009) 33

University of Hanoi 62
University of Rhode Island 46
Unlocking Dyslexia (radio series) 101–102, 104

Vanderbilt, Gloria 59
visual learner 30, 66

Wachenheimer, Ferdinand Friendly 44
Wachenheimer, Terese Friendly 44
WEAN 42, 47–49, 51–52
Wells, Ida B. 99, 108
WGBH 95, 101
White, E.B. 51
World War II 51
Wright, Peter 11

Yale Center for Dyslexia and Creativity 141, 147
Yale University Child Mind Institute 161
Young, Stella 37–39
YouTube 112, 170